MEDICAL MANAGEMENT OF

TYPE 1 DIABETES

FOURTH EDITION

MEDICAL MANAGEMENT OF
TYPE 1 DIABETES

FOURTH EDITION

Bruce W. Bode, MD, Editor

American Diabetes Association.

Cure • Care • Commitment℠

Director, Book Publishing, John Fedor; *Associate Director, Professional Books,* Christine B. Charlip; *Copyeditor/Proofreader,* Wendy M. Martin; *Associate Director, Book Production,* Peggy M. Rote; *Composition,* Circle Graphics; *Cover Design,* Koncept, Inc.; *Printer,* Port City Press

Printed in the United States of America
1 3 5 7 9 10 8 6 4 2

∞ The paper in this publication meets the requirements of the ANSI Standard Z39.48-1992 (permanence of paper).

ADA titles may be purchased for business or promotional use or for special sales. To purchase this book in large quantities, or for custom editions of this book with your logo, contact Lee Romano Sequeira, Special Sales & Promotions, at the address below, or at LRomano@diabetes.org or call 703-299-2046.

American Diabetes Association
1701 North Beauregard Street
Alexandria, Virginia 22311

Library of Congress Cataloging-in-Publication Data

Medical management of type 1 diabetes.—4th ed. / Bruce W. Bode, editor.
  p. ; cm.
  Includes bibliographical references and index.
  ISBN 1-58040-188-0 (pbk. : alk. paper)
   1. Diabetes—Treatment. I. Title: Medical Management of type one diabetes. II. Bode, Bruce W. III. American Diabetes Association.
  [DNLM: 1. Diabetes Mellitus. Insulin-Dependent. WK 810 M4879 2003]
  RC660.M43 2003
  616.4'6206—dc21
                                                                    2003052498

Contents

Special Situations 121

Psychosocial Factors Affecting Adherence, Quality of Life, and Well-Being: Helping Patients Cope   161

Complications 183

A Word About This Guide

*M*edical Management of Type 1 Diabetes is just one of the many books for clinicians published by the American Diabetes Association. Other titles include *Intensive Diabetes Management, The Handbook of Diabetes and Exercise, Medical Management of Type 2 Diabetes, Medical Management of Pregnancy Complicated by Diabetes,* and *Therapy for Diabetes Mellitus and Related Disorders.* These books provide health care professionals with the comprehensive information needed to give the best possible medical care to patients with diabetes.

This book evolved from the *Physician's Guide to Insulin-Dependent (Type I) Diabetes: Diagnosis and Treatment.* During the last decade, much new information has advanced our knowledge of the natural history and pathogenesis of diabetes and its complications. The results of the Diabetes Control and Complications Trial and the long-term follow-up of these patients, as well as other important clinical studies, continue to have major implications for the management of type 1 diabetes. It is clear that blood glucose regulation, proper nutrition, regular exercise, attention to blood pressure and blood lipid levels, and avoidance of smoking are the key elements in the management of type 1 diabetes. No longer are there two modes of diabetes treatment, conventional and intensive. All patients should try to optimize their glucose control through an individualized, flexible treatment regimen—starting at diagnosis—that achieves near-normal glycemia without severe hypoglycemia. The fourth edition of *Medical Management of Type 1 Diabetes* contains the latest clinical practice recommendations of the American Diabetes Association and provides the methodologies to obtain these goals.

The development of *Medical Management of Type 1 Diabetes* was designed to provide state-of-the-art information on these issues. Its publication could not have been possible without the expert guidance of the many contributors of the first, second, and third editions. The book's focus on pathogenesis, diagnosis and classification, patient education and self-management training, medical nutrition therapy, and maintenance of wellness through proper nutrition, exercise, and the prevention and treatment of complications was the work of many experts. I am particularly indebted to the editors who preceded me—Mark A. Sperling, MD; Julio V. Santiago, MD; and Jay S. Skyler, MD—and the many contributors who laid the foundation for the current edition.

With the American Diabetes Association, I trust that you will find this book a useful and practical guide to quality care for patients with type 1 diabetes. Hopefully, it will encourage you to add other American Diabetes Association publications to your library, which can help you manage all your patients with diabetes more effectively, working together toward the goal of optimal glycemic management with avoidance of the devastating complications caused by this disease.

BRUCE W. BODE, MD
Editor

Contributors to the Fourth Edition

EDITOR

Bruce W. Bode, MD
Atlanta Diabetes Associates
Atlanta, Georgia

CONTRIBUTORS

Lloyd P. Aiello, MD, PhD
Joslin Diabetes Center
Boston, Massachusetts

Jerry D. Cavallerano, OD, PhD
Joslin Diabetes Center
Boston, Massachusetts

Paul C. Davidson, MD, FACE
Atlanta Diabetes Associates
Atlanta, Georgia

Sandy Gillespie, MS, RD, LD, CDE
Piedmont Hospital, Diabetes Resource
   Center
Atlanta, Georgia

Charlotte Hayes, MMSc, MS, RD,
   CDE
Diabetes Nutrition and Exercise
   Specialist
Atlanta, Georgia

Lois Jovanovic, MD
Sansum Medical Research Institute
Santa Barbara, California

Phillip A. Lowe, MD
Mayo Clinic
Rochester, Minnesota

Stephen Pastan, MD
Emory University School of Medicine
Piedmont Nephrology and Internal
   Medicine
Atlanta, Georgia

David G. Robertson, MD
Emory University School of Medicine
Atlanta Diabetes Associates
Atlanta, Georgia

Ronald J. Sigal, MD, MPH, FRCPC
University of Ottawa and Ottawa Health
   Research Institute
Ottawa, Canada

R. Dennis Steed, MD, FACE, CDE
Atlanta Diabetes Associates
Atlanta, Georgia

Deborah Young-Hyman, PhD*
National Institute of Child Health and
   Human Development
National Institutes of Health
Bethesda, Maryland

---

*The views in this publication do not necessarily represent the views of the NIH and/or DHHS.

Acknowledgments

The American Diabetes Association gratefully acknowledges the contributions of the following health care professionals and members of the Association's Professional Section to previous editions of this work:

David E. Goldstein, MD; Morey Haymond, MD; Joan Heins, MA, RD, CDE; Julio V. Santiago, MD; Alicia Shiffrin, MD; Donald C. Simonson, MD; Jay S. Skyler, MD; Mark A. Sperling, MD; and Bruce R. Zimmerman, MD.

The Editor thanks the many reviewers who aided in the review and critique of this book, including M. Carol Greenlee, MD; Marci Mann, MD; Linda P. Fredrickson, MA, RN, CDE; Sharon Napolitano; Christian Weyer, MD; and Lauren Beck.

Most of all, the Editor thanks his mentor Paul C. Davidson, MD, FACE; his fellow colleagues; and his patients, who have provided him with invaluable insight on how to best manage people with diabetes.

Diagnosis and Classification/ Pathogenesis

Highlights
Diagnosis and Classification/
Pathogenesis

DIAGNOSIS AND CLASSIFICATION

■ Diabetes encompasses a wide clinical spectrum. The vast majority of cases of diabetes fall into two broad etiopathogenetic categories:

- type 1 diabetes, the cause of which is an absolute deficiency of insulin secretion
- type 2 diabetes, the cause of which is a combination of resistance to insulin action and an inadequate compensatory insulin secretory response

■ Indications for diagnostic testing include

- positive screening test results
- obvious signs and symptoms of diabetes mellitus (polydipsia, polyuria, polyphagia, weight loss)
- an incomplete clinical picture, such as glucosuria or equivocal elevation of random plasma glucose level

■ When diabetes is fully evolved, fasting plasma glucose levels exceed 126 mg/dl (>7.0 mmol/l), and random plasma glucose levels exceed 200 mg/dl (>11.1 mmol/l).

■ Approximately 1 in every 400–500 children and adolescents has type 1 diabetes. Incidence is similar in males and females, lower in African Americans than whites, and markedly less common in Hispanics, Asian Americans, and American Indians.

■ At presentation, patients with type 1 diabetes can be at any age, are lean, and often have experienced significant weight loss, polyuria, and polydipsia before presentation. The oral glucose tolerance test is rarely needed to diagnose type 1 diabetes. Delayed diagnosis is a serious, sometimes fatal, problem, especially among younger children.

■ Approximately 40% of children <2 yr old present in coma, and of these, ~5% die.

■ Type 1 diabetes can develop at any age and is sometimes mistaken for type 2 diabetes among older patients.

PATHOGENESIS

■ The primary defect in type 1 diabetes is inadequate insulin secretion by pancreatic β-cells.

■ Genetic predisposition clearly plays a role in development of type 1 diabetes. However, environmental factors may be involved in initiating β-cell destruction, which is carried out by an autoimmune process not completely understood.

■ Detectable abnormalities of insulin secretion may be preceded by months to years of β-cell destruction, noted by the presence of antibodies to islet cell components.

■ Fasting hyperglycemia occurs when β-cell mass is reduced by 80–90%. Typical symptoms of diabetes, i.e., polyuria, polydipsia, and weight loss, appear once hyperglycemia exceeds the renal threshold of ~180 mg/dl (~10.0 mmol/l) glucose.

■ Sometime after diagnosis and correction of acute metabolic abnormalities, some individuals experience a "honeymoon phase," a temporary period when the need for exogenous insulin is diminished or absent.

■ Within 5–10 yr after clinical presentation, β-cell loss is complete; at this point, insulin deficiency is absolute, and circulating islet cell antibodies can no longer be detected.

Diagnosis and Classification/ Pathogenesis

DIAGNOSIS AND CLASSIFICATION

Diabetes mellitus is a chronic disorder that is *1*) characterized by hyperglycemia, *2*) associated with major abnormalities in carbohydrate, fat, and protein metabolism, and *3*) accompanied by a marked propensity to develop relatively specific forms of renal, ocular, neurologic, and premature cardiovascular diseases. Diabetes encompasses a wide clinical spectrum. The vast majority of cases of diabetes fall into two broad etiopathogenetic categories:

- type 1 diabetes, the cause of which is an absolute deficiency of insulin secretion
- type 2 diabetes, the cause of which is a combination of resistance to insulin action and an inadequate compensatory insulin secretory response

Diabetes may also occur because of specific genetic defects and secondary to a number of conditions and syndromes, including diseases of the pancreas, several endocrinopathies, and use of certain drugs.

Although type 1 diabetes accounts for ~5–10% of all diagnosed cases of diabetes, its immediate risks and stringent acute treatment requirements demand rapid recognition, diagnosis, and management. This chapter explores characteristics that differentiate type 1 diabetes from other forms of diabetes, discusses criteria for correct diagnosis, and illustrates various clinical presentations.

CRITERIA FOR DIAGNOSIS

Diabetes is diagnosed when the fasting plasma glucose concentration exceeds 126 mg/dl (7.0 mmol/l) and/or random plasma glucose levels exceed 200 mg/dl (11.1 mmol/l) on more than one occasion with or without overt symptoms of diabetes. The clinical signs and/or symptoms that accompany diabetes are polyuria, polydipsia, fatigue, polyphagia, weight loss, or blurred vision and persistent hyperglycemia. In the young child or infant, these signs or symptoms are frequently missed until the child presents with unexplained dehydration, acidosis, and/or a severe candidal diaper rash. Under the above circumstances, an oral glucose tolerance test (OGTT) is not needed, and its use is contraindicated (Table 1.1). In fact, an OGTT is rarely needed to diagnose type 1 diabetes.

Although not considered diagnostic, an elevated glycated hemoglobin (A1C) may confirm the presence of significant preexisting hyperglycemia (barring the presence of a hemoglobin variant). Pre-diabetes (previously known as impaired

---

Table 1.1 Criteria for Diagnosis of Diabetes Mellitus in Nonpregnant Adults

Diagnosis of diabetes mellitus in nonpregnant adults should be restricted to those who have one of the following:

- Symptoms of diabetes plus casual plasma glucose concentration ≥200 mg/dl (11.1 mmol/l). The classic symptoms of diabetes include polyuria, polydipsia, and unexplained weight loss. Casual refers to any time of day without regard to time since last meal.

  or

- Fasting plasma glucose ≥126 mg/dl (7.0 mmol/l). Fasting is defined as no caloric intake for at least 8 h.

  or

- 2-h plasma glucose ≥200 mg/dl (11.1 mmol/l) during an oral glucose tolerance test (OGTT).* The test should be performed using a glucose load containing the equivalent of 75 g anhydrous glucose dissolved in water.

In the absence of unequivocal hyperglycemia with acute metabolic decompensation, these criteria should be confirmed by repeat testing on a different day.

*An OGTT is rarely needed to diagnose type 1 diabetes and is not recommended for routine clinical use.

---

glucose tolerance or impaired fasting glucose) as distinguished from diabetes mellitus, refers to abnormal plasma glucose values that do not meet the established criteria to diagnose diabetes. Because the diagnosis of diabetes has profound effects on an individual's ability to obtain affordable health care and life insurance and may affect his or her vocational careers, great care should be taken in not labeling an individual with pre-diabetes as having diabetes.

RISK OF DEVELOPING TYPE 1 DIABETES

Although type 1 diabetes is much less common in the general population than type 2 diabetes, type 1 diabetes is by no means rare among children and young adults. In the US, approximately 1 in every 400–500 children and adolescents has type 1 diabetes. It is one of the most common childhood diseases, with a much higher incidence rate than many other chronic childhood diseases, such as cystic fibrosis, juvenile rheumatoid arthritis, nephrotic syndrome, muscular dystrophy, or leukemia. About 150,000 people under age 20, and 400,000 people age ≥20, have type 1 diabetes.

The annual incidence of type 1 diabetes decreases after age 20. Incidence is similar in men and women; it is lower in African Americans, Hispanics, Asian Americans, and American Indians than in whites.

The risk of diabetes to family members of an individual with type 1 diabetes is significantly higher compared with the general population. The statistical risk of a family member developing type 1 diabetes is linked to the genetic similarities of the family members. For example, when one identical twin develops diabetes, the risk to the other twin is 25–50%. This is in contrast to a 0.4% risk in the general population, a 15% risk in a human leukocyte antigen (HLA)–identical sibling, and a 1% risk in an HLA-nonidentical sibling.

DISTINGUISHING TYPE 1 DIABETES FROM OTHER FORMS

Type 1 Diabetes

Type 1 diabetes can develop at any age. Although more cases are diagnosed before the patient is 30 yr old, it also occurs in older individuals. Because patients with type 1 diabetes are insulinopenic, insulin therapy is essential to prevent rapid and severe dehydration, catabolism, ketoacidosis, and death (Table 1.2). Most patients are lean and have experienced significant weight loss, polyuria, polydipsia, and fatigue before presentation. At presentation, they often have significant elevations of A1C, providing evidence of weeks, if not months, of hyperglycemia. In addition, 90–95% have circulating antibodies directed against one or more islet cell components.

Table 1.2 Distinguishing Characteristics of the Major Types of Diabetes Mellitus

Clinical Classes

Type 1 diabetes
  β-Cell destruction, usually leading to absolute insulin deficiency

Type 2 diabetes
  Ranging from predominantly insulin resistance with relative insulin deficiency to predominantly an insulin secretory defect with insulin resistance

Secondary and other types of diabetes

Gestational diabetes mellitus

Distinguishing Characteristics

Type 1 diabetes patients may be of any age, are not usually obese, and often have abrupt onset of signs and symptoms with insulinopenia before age 30. These patients are often strongly positive for ketones in conjunction with hyperglycemia and are eventually dependent on insulin therapy to prevent ketoacidosis and to sustain life.

Type 2 diabetes patients usually are >30 yr old at diagnosis, obese, and have relatively few classic symptoms. They are not prone to ketoacidosis except during periods of stress. Although not dependent on exogenous insulin for survival, they may require it for adequate control of hyperglycemia.

Patients with secondary and other types of diabetes mellitus have certain associated conditions or syndromes (see Table 1.3).

Patients with gestational diabetes mellitus have onset or discovery of glucose intolerance during pregnancy.

Type 2 Diabetes

In contrast, patients with type 2 diabetes are not prone to develop ketoacidosis unless severely stressed physiologically, are generally but not always obese, may be asymptomatic or only mildly symptomatic, and usually have a family history of diabetes. Type 2 diabetes is said to generally present after age 30, but an increasing number of obese adolescents and young adults have been presenting with type 2 diabetes, especially among African Americans, Native Americans, and Hispanics. Note that some of these patients present in ketoacidosis, which can be fatal.

Patients with type 2 diabetes are not absolutely dependent on exogenous insulin for survival, although insulin therapy is often used to lower blood glucose levels (Table 1.2).

Genetic Defects Presenting with Childhood Onset

Several forms of diabetes are associated with monogenetic defects in β-cell function. These forms of diabetes are frequently characterized by onset of mild hyperglycemia at an early age, generally before age 25. They were formerly referred to as maturity-onset diabetes of the young (MODY), and they are characterized by impaired insulin secretion with minimal or no defects in insulin action. They are inherited in an autosomal-dominant pattern. Abnormalities at three genetic loci on different chromosomes have been identified to date:

- mutations on chromosome 12 in the hepatic transcription factor hepatocyte nuclear factor (HNF)-1α
- mutations on chromosome 7p in the glucokinase gene
- mutation on chromosome 20q in the hepatic transcription factor HNF-4α gene

There also are unusual causes of diabetes that result from genetically determined abnormalities of insulin action. Leprechaunism and the Rabson-Mendenhall syndrome are two pediatric syndromes that have mutations in the insulin receptor gene with subsequent alterations in insulin receptor function and extreme insulin resistance. The former has characteristic facial features and is usually fatal in infancy, whereas the latter is associated with abnormalities of teeth and nails and pineal gland hyperplasia.

Not Quite Type 1 or Type 2 Diabetes

Some patients are difficult to categorize as having type 1 or type 2 diabetes. The routinely available laboratory tests that help differentiate between the two types are serum C-peptide levels and measurements of various antibodies to islet cell components. Almost all patients with long-term type 1 diabetes will have C-peptide values below the lower limit of normal for that assay method, with most being undetectable. However, C-peptide levels in recently diagnosed type 1 diabetes are often in normal range and decline over the next several months to years after diagnosis.

Absent availability of measurement of antibodies or C-peptide, if a patient is <30 yr old, not obese, and has signs and symptoms of diabetes mellitus and an elevated fasting plasma glucose, the physician should assume type 1 diabetes and treat with insulin. The presence of moderate ketonuria with hyperglycemia in an otherwise unstressed individual strongly supports a diagnosis of type 1 diabetes, whereas the absence or modest ketonuria is of no diagnostic value.

Clinicians should also be aware that some cases presenting as type 2 diabetes subsequently may be discovered to be type 1 diabetes. In these individuals, antibodies to islet cell components may indicate the eventual need for insulin therapy. These patients are usually lean, and their insulin requirements increase as they develop manifestations of complete insulin deficiency. In contrast, occasionally some adolescents and young adults who present with typical signs and symptoms of type 1 diabetes later require insulin treatment only intermittently. Table 1.3 illustrates specific conditions often associated with other forms of diabetes and glucose intolerance. Further studies are required to determine the pathophysiology of these conditions.

Table 1.3 Other Specific Types of Diabetes

Genetic Defects of β-Cell Function

Examples: chromosome 12–HNF-1α (formerly MODY 3); chromosome 7–glucokinase (formerly MODY 2); chromosome 20–HNF-4α (formerly MODY 1); mitochondrial DNA

Genetic Defects in Insulin Action

Examples: type A insulin resistance, leprechaunism, Rabson-Mendenhall syndrome, lipoatrophic diabetes

Diseases of the Exocrine Pancreas

Examples: pancreatitis, trauma or pancreatectomy, neoplasia, cystic fibrosis, hemochromatosis, fibrocalculous pancreatopathy

Endocrinopathies

Examples: acromegaly, Cushing's syndrome, glucagonoma, pheochromocytoma, hyperthyroidism, somatostatinoma, aldosteronoma

Drug- or Chemical-Induced Diabetes

Examples: Vacor, pentamidine, nicotinic acid, glucocorticoids, thyroid hormone, diazoxide, β-adrenergic agonists, thiazides, Dilantin, interferon-α

Infections

Examples: congenital rubella, cytomegalovirus

Uncommon Forms of Immune-Mediated Diabetes

Examples: "stiff man" syndrome, anti-insulin receptor antibodies

Genetic Syndromes Sometimes Associated with Diabetes

Examples: Down's syndrome, Klinefelter's syndrome, Turner's syndrome, Wolfram's syndrome, Friedreich's ataxia, Huntington's chorea, Lawrence-Moon-Bardet-Biedl syndrome, myotonic dystrophy, porphyria, Prader-Willi syndrome

CLINICAL PRESENTATION OF TYPE 1 DIABETES

The presentation of type 1 diabetes covers a broad range, from mild nonspecific symptoms or no symptoms to coma. In children, correct diagnosis is often delayed because polyuria is incorrectly attributed to urinary tract infection or enuresis; anorexia rather than polyphagia may occur; and fatigue, irritability, weight loss, deterioration of school performance, and secondary enuresis are ascribed to emotional problems. In some cases, "failure to thrive" may be an overlooked indication of diabetes in a young child.

Fewer patients with previously undiagnosed type 1 diabetes are presenting in severe diabetic ketoacidosis than in the past, and >75% of cases are diagnosed within 1 mo of onset of symptoms. Nevertheless, delayed diagnosis continues to be a serious and occasionally fatal problem, especially among younger children. The symptoms of polyuria are less obvious in the young child and are frequently missed until metabolic decompensation has occurred. These very young children frequently present with severe dehydration, metabolic acidosis, and a clinical history that is inconsistent with the severity of their clinical appearance, e.g., absence of diarrhea or significant vomiting. Because of the delay in the diagnosis of the younger child, the frequency of coma as a presenting feature is considerably greater in children <2 yr of age than in older children, adolescents, and adults. In young adults, the presentation is often less acute, although an absolute requirement for insulin becomes evident with time.

CONCLUSION

Patients with type 1 diabetes are dependent on insulin for as long as they live. Any lean individual <30 yr of age with typical signs and symptoms of hyperglycemia accompanied by weight loss should be assumed to have type 1 diabetes. A high index of suspicion is needed to diagnose diabetes in very young children or elderly patients.

BIBLIOGRAPHY

American Diabetes Association: Report of the Expert Committee on the Diagnosis and Classification of Diabetes Mellitus. *Diabetes Care* 26 (Suppl. 1): S5–S20, 2003

Rosenbloom AL, Silverstein JK: *Type 2 Diabetes in Children and Adolescents.* Alexandria, VA, American Diabetes Association, 2003

PATHOGENESIS

The primary defect in type 1 diabetes mellitus is decreased insulin secretion by pancreatic β-cells. This single defect accounts for the hyperglycemia, polyuria, polydipsia, weight loss, dehydration, electrolyte disturbance, and ketoacidosis observed in patients presenting for the first time with type 1 diabetes. The capacity of normal pancreatic β-cells to secrete insulin is far in excess of that normally needed to control carbohydrate, fat, and protein metabolism. As a result, clinical onset is preceded by an extensive asymptomatic period during which β-cells are inexorably destroyed. The evolving process of β-cell destruction reaches a point where insufficient insulin is secreted to maintain normal plasma glucose concentrations, which causes the broadly predictable abnormalities in carbohydrate, fat, and protein metabolism characterizing the uncontrolled diabetic condition.

Most patients with type 1 diabetes have immune-mediated diabetes mellitus. This form of diabetes results from a cellular-mediated autoimmune destruction of the β-cells of the pancreas. Most of the discussion in this section deals with this form of type 1 diabetes—immune-mediated diabetes mellitus. However, some forms of type 1 diabetes have no evidence of autoimmunity or other known etiology and are labeled "idiopathic." Some of these patients have permanent insulinopenia and are prone to ketoacidosis. Although only a minority of patients with type 1 diabetes fall into the idiopathic category, of those who do, most are of African or Asian origin. Individuals with this form of diabetes often suffer from episodic ketoacidosis and exhibit varying degrees of insulin deficiency between episodes. This form of diabetes is strongly inherited, lacks immunological evidence for β-cell autoimmunity, and is not HLA associated. An absolute requirement for insulin replacement therapy in affected patients may come and go.

PATHOPHYSIOLOGY OF THE CLINICAL ONSET OF TYPE 1 DIABETES

Insulin is the primary hormone that suppresses hepatic glucose production, lipolysis, and proteolysis. It increases the transport of glucose into adipocytes and myocytes and stimulates glycogen synthesis. In the presence of adequate plasma amino acids, insulin maintains or perhaps stimulates whole-body protein anabolism. As such, insulin is the primary hormone of anabolism of meal-derived nutrients (Table 1.4).

In the postabsorptive state, the plasma concentration of glucose is maintained in a narrow range (80–95 mg/dl [4.4–5.3 mmol/l]) by precise regulation of hepatic glucose release and peripheral glucose utilization.

Basal plasma insulin concentrations maintain hepatic glucose release at a rate of 1.9–2.1 mg/kg/min (10–12 μmol/l/kg/min). This is of critical importance to provide adequate glucose for the brain, which accounts for nearly 50% of total glucose utilization under these conditions. With prolonged fasting, the plasma insulin concentration decreases even further, permitting increased mobilization of free fatty acids (FFAs). The resulting increase in circulating FFA concentration drives hepatic ketogenesis, which results in ketosis. Increased availability of plasma FFAs, β-hydroxybutyrate, and acetoacetate provides alternative metabolic

Table 1.4 Physiological Effects of High- Versus Low-Insulin States

	High-Insulin (Fed) State	Low-Insulin (Fasted) State
Liver	Glucose uptake Glycogen synthesis Lipogenesis Absent ketogenesis Absent gluconeogenesis	Glucose production Glycogenolysis Absent lipogenesis Ketogenesis Gluconeogenesis
Muscle	Glucose uptake Glucose oxidation Glycogen synthesis Sustained protein synthesis	Absent glucose uptake Fatty acid, ketone oxidation Glycogenolysis Proteolysis and amino acid release
Adipose tissue	Glucose uptake Lipid synthesis Triglyceride uptake	Absent glucose uptake Lipolysis and fatty acid release Absent triglyceride uptake

fuels to glucose and reduces the rates of glucose utilization by peripheral tissues and brain.

After ingestion of a mixed meal, nearly 85% of ingested glucose enters the systemic circulation. The increasing arterial glucose concentration stimulates the secretion of insulin into the portal vein. About half of the secreted insulin is extracted by the liver, which signals the suppression of hepatic glucose release. The unextracted insulin enters the systemic circulation, where it stimulates glucose uptake, primarily by muscle, and decreases lipolysis and proteolysis. This facilitates a continuous entry of glucose into the systemic circulation by permitting a switch from endogenous glucose production to exogenous glucose. As dietary glucose entry decreases with the absorption of the meal-derived carbohydrate, plasma glucose decreases, as does the secretion and plasma concentration of insulin. When plasma glucose reaches or even falls slightly below basal concentrations, hepatic glucose production is again increased by both the decrease in plasma insulin and by an increase in plasma glucagon concentration (Table 1.4).

PROGRESSION OF METABOLIC ABNORMALITIES DURING ONSET

The insulin secretory reserves of the normal pancreas are considerable. Therefore, individuals destined to develop type 1 diabetes go through a variable interval of months to years of autoimmune β-cell destruction before abnormalities in insulin secretion or glucose metabolism can be detected (Fig. 1.1).

The earliest detectable abnormality in insulin secretion is a progressive reduction of the immediate (first-phase) plasma insulin response during intravenous glucose tolerance testing. This impairment alone has little deleterious effect on overall glucose homeostasis: fasting plasma glucose concentrations remain normal, and the response to an OGTT is virtually unimpaired. At this stage of the

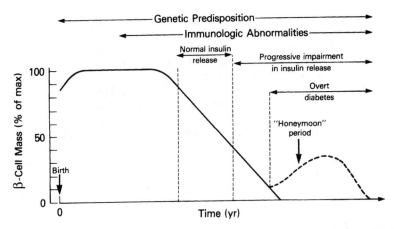

Figure 1.1 Proposed scheme of natural history of β-cell defect. Timing of trigger in relation to immunologic abnormalities is unknown. Note that overt diabetes is not apparent until insulin secretory reserves are <10–20% of normal.

disease, most affected individuals have circulating antibodies to islet cell components, islet cell antibodies (ICAs), including antibodies to their own insulin, and to other islet cell antigens (e.g., glutamic acid decarboxylase [GAD] and islet tyrosine phosphatases known as IA2 and IA2β). These are markers of an ongoing autoimmune process that eventuates in type 1 diabetes. The presence of significant titers of antibodies, or the combination of several circulating antibodies, together with impaired first-phase insulin secretion, appears predictive of type 1 diabetes (Fig. 1.1).

CLINICAL ONSET OF DIABETIC SYMPTOMS AND METABOLIC DECOMPENSATION

When ongoing destruction has reduced β-cell mass by 80–90%, the individual's insulin secretory capacity becomes insufficient to normally regulate hepatic glucose production (Fig. 1.1). Initially, only postprandial hyperglycemia occurs, reflecting a failure to adequately suppress hepatic glucose production during meal absorption together with some decrease in peripheral glucose utilization. But as insulin secretion is further compromised, progressive fasting hyperglycemia occurs as a result of increased basal hepatic glucose production and decreased glucose uptake by peripheral tissue. Hyperglycemia per se may further compromise glucose utilization by reducing the number and/or activity of glucose transporters available on both insulin-dependent and non–insulin-dependent tissues, a phenomenon known as "glucose toxicity."

When the plasma glucose concentration exceeds the renal threshold of ~180 mg/dl (10.0 mmol/1), glucosuria results in an osmotic diuresis, generating the classic symptoms of polyuria and a compensatory polydipsia. If untreated, the symptoms usually progress as the hyperglycemia and glucosuria increase. With evolving insulin deficiency, weight loss occurs as body fat and protein stores are reduced because of increased rates of lipolysis and proteolysis. With the super-imposed metabolic abnormalities of diabetes itself or with a minor viral or bacterial infection, plasma concentrations of glucagon, growth hormone, epi-nephrine, and cortisol increase. These hormones antagonize insulin's effect, fur-ther promoting hepatic glucose production (by stimulating both glycogenolysis and gluconeogenesis), lipolysis, ketogenesis, and proteolysis. As long as fluid intake is sufficient to offset the fluid losses resulting from the combined diuresis of both glucosuria and ketonuria, some individuals can remain compensated for weeks, if not months. Should the individual be unable to consume adequate amounts of fluid as a result of nausea from the ketosis or because of an intercur-rent illness, rapid and severe losses of both intra- and extracellular fluid and elec-trolytes can ensue and, in the course of hours, lead to a clinical presentation of severe ketoacidosis.

Honeymoon Phase

At initial presentation with symptomatic hyperglycemia and/or ketosis, circu-lating insulin concentrations are low, and there is no significant β-cell response to any of the usual insulin secretagogues. Initially, exogenous insulin requirements are relatively large, due not only to the reduced insulin secretion but also to insulin resistance.

After the correction of the hyperglycemia, metabolic acidosis, and ketosis, endogenous insulin secretion recovers (Fig. 1.1). During this time, exogenous insulin requirements may decrease dramatically. During the honeymoon period, which may last for up to 1 yr or longer, good metabolic control may be easily achieved with either conventional or intensive insulin therapy. The need for increasing exogenous insulin replacement is inevitable and should always be antic-ipated. Recent evidence from the Diabetes Control and Complications Trial follow-up cohort suggests that intensive insulin therapy from early diagnosis pro-longs C-peptide secretion and thus creates less major hypoglycemia and less microvascular complications 10 yr after diagnosis. As a result, intensive insulin therapy with strict attention to diet and self-monitoring of blood glucose should be initiated at diagnosis and maintained.

Finally, within 5 yr for children and 10 yr after clinical presentation regardless of age at presentation, β-cell destruction is essentially complete. At this point, insulin deficiency is usually absolute.

Immune Therapy

The role of several immune therapies in preserving the remaining β-cells before metabolic decompensation has been studied in individuals at the clinical onset of diabetes (prolonged, asymptomatic phase). Early therapeutic attempts centered mainly on general immune suppression. Although effective in small pilot studies in prolonging the honeymoon period or delaying the onset of overt type 1 diabetes, none resulted in permanent remission. Two recent large, multicenter intervention trials involving either low-dose insulin therapy (Diabetes Prevention Trial 1 [DPT-1]) or nicotinamide (ENDIT Trial) in the pre–type 1 diabetes state showed no benefit in delaying or preventing the onset of type 1 diabetes. A second arm of the DPT-1 using oral insulin in those deemed to be of moderate risk (25–50% risk) of developing diabetes also showed no benefit.

Newer approaches are being developed and investigated to resume a state of immune tolerance to islet cells and/or to abrogate immune effects (e.g., free radical generation) in individuals with pre–type 1 diabetes. These intervention trials offer an opportunity to preserve a significant mass of β-cells and potentially prevent or delay overt diabetes. Potential therapeutic modalities must be approached with caution and should be utilized only in conjunction with carefully defined scientific studies.

GENETICS AND IMMUNOLOGY OF TYPE 1 DIABETES

Type 1 diabetes is a genetically influenced and immunologically mediated disease with a prolonged asymptomatic phase (pre–type 1 diabetes), which eventually results in progressive β-cell destruction, insulin deficiency, and overt clinical symptoms. The identity of the initiating event(s) remains speculative.

The familial predisposition to type 1 diabetes has long been known. A specific mode of genetic transmission has not been established. Predisposition to type 1 diabetes is inherited as a heterogeneous multigenic trait with low penetrance and gender biases. There is a higher concordance rate for type 1 diabetes in monozygotic twins (25–50%) than in dizygotic twins (6%). The empirical risk of type 1 diabetes is increased in first-degree relatives of probands with the disease (Table 1.5). In the US, among whites, the overall risk is 0.2–0.4%. However, in siblings of probands with type 1 diabetes, the risk is about 5%, whereas offspring of parents with diabetes have a 3% risk if the mother has the disease and a 6% risk if the father has the disease (Table 1.5).

About 40–50% of the genetic predisposition to type 1 diabetes is conferred by genes on the short arm of chromosome 6, either within or in close proximity to the Class II HLA region of the major histocompatibility complex (MHC). At least

Table 1.5 Approximate Familial Risk of Type 1 Diabetes

Relationship to Proband	Risk (%)
Sibling	6
Identical twin	25–50
HLA	
Identical	15
Haploidentical	6
Nonidentical	1
Father	6
Mother	3
Offspring	5
General population	0.3–0.4

Adapted from Muir A, Schatz DA, Maclaren NK: The pathogenesis, prediction, and prevention of insulin-dependent diabetes mellitus. *Endocrin Metab Clin North Am* 21:199–219, 1992.

11 other loci have been suggested to be involved, with the largest contribution (about 10% of the genetic predisposition) being accounted for by the flanking region of the insulin gene on chromosome 11.

The Class II MHC DR and DQ molecules are comprised of an α- and a β-chain, which present processed antigen to T-cells. The relationship between type 1 diabetes and specific MHC Class II region alleles is complex. There is a strong positive relationship with HLA-DR3 and -DR4 and a strong negative relationship with -DR2. Indeed, more than 90% of whites with type 1 diabetes are HLA-DR3 and/or -DR4. There is an even stronger relationship of type 1 diabetes when DQ loci (DQα and DQβ) are considered together with DR loci, i.e., the predisposition to type 1 diabetes in whites is associated with HLA-DR3, DQB1*0201 and with HLA-DR4,DQB1*0302, with the strongest association being the DQα-DQβ combination DQA1*0501-DQB1*0302. Other DQ alleles appear to confer protection from type 1 diabetes, e.g., DQA1*0201-DQB1*0602 provides protection even in the presence of DQ susceptibility alleles. This suggests that protection is dominant over susceptibility. Because Class II MHC genes regulate the immune response, the susceptibility and protective alleles could be involved differentially in antigen presentation of peptides that establish and maintain tolerance or influence the immune response.

Thus, there are genes that confer susceptibility or predisposition to the disease and genes that confer protection against development of the disease. Nevertheless, it remains unclear what are the genetic factors that confer susceptibility or, by contrast, that confer protection.

Autoantibodies and Autoantigens

The identification of circulating autoantibodies to islet cell components in diabetic and subsequently in nondiabetic first-degree relatives has made it possible to detect the preclinical disease. Numerous circulating antibodies have been identified, including cytoplasmic ICAs detected by immunofluorescence, insulin autoantibodies (IAAs), antibodies directed against the enzyme GAD, antibodies against islet tyrosine phosphatase (known as IA2 and IA2β), and several others. Most (>90%) newly diagnosed patients with type 1 diabetes have one or another of these circulating antibodies as do 3.5–4% of unaffected first-degree relatives. This latter group of antibody-positive individuals is at increased risk for developing type 1 diabetes. The presence of two or more antibodies, together with decreased first-phase insulin secretion, is predictive of increased risk of type 1 diabetes within 5 yr.

These autoantibodies generally are not thought to mediate β-cell destruction by humoral mechanisms. Rather, it is likely that as β-cells are destroyed, multiple antigens are exposed to the immune system, with generation of antibodies directed against these components. Thus, these antibodies are markers of immune activity or of β-cell damage and herald the disease process several years before overt clinical hyperglycemia. As β-cell function is lost and "total" diabetes evolves, antibodies tend to decrease in titer and/or disappear.

Many patients with type 1 diabetes have nonpancreatic organ-specific autoantibodies (e.g., thyroid, gastric parietal cells, and less often, adrenal). Although Hashimoto's thyroiditis is the most common autoimmune disorder associated with type 1 diabetes, the range of organ involvement can vary from none to severe polyglandular failure.

Screening and Intervention Trials

Humoral autoantibodies allow for the identification of individuals who are at high risk for developing type 1 diabetes, and they play a role in experimental therapeutic trials directed at the preservation of islet cell function. Screening for immunologic markers of type 1 diabetes in any population outside the context of defined research studies is discouraged. Screening of high-risk individuals (e.g., first-degree relatives of someone with type 1 diabetes) should be encouraged, provided that individuals who screen positive are referred to centers participating in cooperative intervention studies or other scientific investigations using appropriate techniques. All subjects who are screened but do not enter a study should be counseled about their risk of developing diabetes, and follow-up should be offered.

Cell-Mediated Immunologic Dysfunction

The existence of insulitis (lymphocytic infiltration of the pancreas by mononuclear cells) has been known for decades and was the earliest evidence for the autoimmune nature of type 1 diabetes. There is evidence of a role for both T- and B-cells as well as lymphokines in the pathophysiology of the β-cell destruction in both human and animal models. However, type 1 diabetes in most animal models is considered a cell-mediated disease because adoptive transfer occurs with T-cells but not with autoantibody transfer. Therapies directed against T-cells are more successful than antibody-depleting treatments such as plasmapheresis.

Environmental Triggers

The concordance rate of diabetes of identical twins suggests that environmental factors may be important in the pathogenesis of type 1 diabetes. Viral infections, e.g., Coxsackie B4 and congenital rubella, have been inconsistently implicated as triggers for the immunologic process. Exposure to substances toxic to the β-cells accounts for only a very small number of cases. Prolonged breastfeeding is reported to lower the incidence rates for type 1 diabetes. Little direct evidence exists to link any specific factor(s) to triggering autoimmune destruction of the β-cells in type 1 diabetes in humans.

CONCLUSION

Individuals who are genetically or otherwise predisposed to develop type 1 diabetes eventually demonstrate near total failure of insulin secretion as the result of an immunologically mediated progressive destruction of β-cell mass. The emergence of insulinopenia is associated with several intracellular abnormalities in both liver and muscle tissue, leading to excessive hepatic glucose production, decreased muscle glucose uptake, frank glucose intolerance, and if untreated, ketoacidosis. Because insulin deficiency is primary, patients are dependent on exogenous insulin for life.

BIBLIOGRAPHY

American Diabetes Association: Report of the Expert Committee on the Diagnosis and Classification of Diabetes Mellitus. *Diabetes Care* 26 (Suppl. 1):S5–S20, 2003

American Diabetes Association: Prevention of type 1 diabetes mellitus (Position Statement). *Diabetes Care* 26 (Suppl. 1):S140, 2003

Atkinson MA, Maclaren NK: The pathogenesis of insulin-dependent diabetes mellitus. *N Engl J Med* 331:1428–1436, 1994

Bach JF: Insulin-dependent diabetes mellitus as an autoimmune disease. *Endocr Rev* 15:516–542, 1994

Genuth SM: Diabetic ketoacidosis and hyperglycemic hyperosmolar coma. *Curr Ther Endocrinol Metab* 6:438–447, 1997

Nepom GT: Immunogenetics and IDDM. *Diabetes Reviews* 1:93–103, 1993

Palmer JP: Predicting IDDM: use of humoral markers: autoantigens of IDDM. *Diabetes Reviews* 1:104–116, 1993

Rabinovitch A: Immunoregulatory and cytokine imbalances in the pathogenesis of IDDM: therapeutic intervention by immunostimulation? *Diabetes* 43:613–621, 1994

Rossini AA, Greiner DL, Friedman HP, Mordes JP: Immunopathogenesis of diabetes mellitus. *Diabetes Reviews* 1:43–75, 1993

Skyler JS, Marks JB: Immune intervention in type I diabetes mellitus. *Diabetes Reviews* 1:15–42, 1993

Thai AC, Eisenbarth GS: Natural history of IDDM: autoantigens of IDDM. *Diabetes Reviews* 1:1–14, 1993

Type 1 Diabetes Study Group: Effects of insulin in relatives of patients with type 1 diabetes. *N Engl J Med* 346:1685–1691, 2002

Writing Team for the Diabetes Control and Complications Trial/Epidemiology of Diabetes Interventions and Complications Research Group: Effect of intensive therapy on the microvascular complications of type 1 diabetes mellitus. *JAMA* 287:2563–2569, 2002

Diabetes Standards and Education

Highlights
Diabetes Standards
and Education

PHILOSOPHY AND GOALS

■ Three factors that strongly influence treatment are

- the diabetes management team's treatment philosophy, including beliefs regarding glycemic control and complications
- the patient's self-care attitudes and abilities
- physician-patient alignment of goals

■ The primary goals of treatment are to

- achieve optimal glycemic goals with a flexible, individualized diabetes management plan
- avoid severe hypoglycemia, symptomatic hyperglycemia, and ketoacidosis
- promote and maintain day-to-day clinical and psychological well-being
- promote normal growth and development in children

■ Results from the Diabetes Control and Complications Trial demonstrated a link between glycemic control and development of diabetic complications.

■ The physician and patient must set treatment goals together with the diabetes management team and family. Glycemic goals should be set as close to optimal as possible given the patient's abilities and presence of risk factors.

■ Initial and long-term clinical goals are presented in Clinical Goals. They focus on

- metabolic stabilization
- restoration and maintenance of desirable body weight
- elimination of hyperglycemic symptoms

DIABETES SELF-MANAGEMENT EDUCATION

■ The goal of diabetes self-management education is to provide patients with the knowledge, skills, and motivation to incorporate diabetes self-management into their daily life. To meet this goal, diabetes education must provide

- teaching of information needed for diabetes self-management
- training in skills needed for treatment procedures

- guidance on devising methods to fit the treatment regimen into the individual's lifestyle
- counseling on reconciling diabetes care and the individual's view of quality of life

■ Diabetes self-management education is a planned process that includes

- assessment to identify the patient's individual education needs
- planning specific education strategies
- implementation and documentation of education
- evaluation of effectiveness

To be effective, patient education must be individualized, should be provided in a team approach to diabetes care, and needs to continue across the life span of the individual with diabetes.

■ Newly diagnosed patients with type 1 diabetes need to learn the basic skills that will enable them to implement their treatment regimen at home. Initial education should focus on teaching survival skills, with more in-depth information and additional topics added after the patient has had time to adjust to diabetes self-management. Written patient guidelines for detecting and treating hypoglycemia and for managing mild illnesses reinforce self-management skills that are not routinely needed.

■ Patient education is essential for management of type 1 diabetes. Therefore, physicians who treat type 1 diabetes patients need to provide diabetes self-management training. Physicians can incorporate diabetes patient education in their clinical practice by

- hiring diabetes educators
- developing a team relationship with diabetes educators working in the community
- referring patients to diabetes education programs recognized by the American Diabetes Association as meeting the National Standards for Diabetes Self-Management Education

Diabetes Standards
and Education

PHILOSOPHY AND GOALS

Type 1 diabetes mellitus is a chronic disease in which the goals and attitudes of the diabetes management team together with those of the patient are paramount in determining management and outcome. The diabetes management team comprises a consortium that includes the endocrinologist or diabetes specialist, nurse, dietitian, social worker, mental health professional, and medical specialists. Three factors that strongly influence treatment are

- the diabetes management team's treatment philosophy, including beliefs regarding glycemic control and complications
- the patient's self-care attitudes and abilities
- physician-patient congruence of goals

The primary goals of treatment are *1*) to promote and maintain day-to-day clinical and psychological well-being; *2*) to avoid severe hypoglycemia, symptomatic hyperglycemia, and ketoacidosis; and *3*) to promote normal growth and development in children. The secondary goal of treatment is to provide the patient with the necessary tools to achieve the best possible glycemic control to prevent, delay, or arrest the micro- and macrovascular complications while minimizing hypoglycemia and excess weight gain. The primary goals are clearly achievable at reasonable degrees of cost, inconvenience, and risk; the secondary goal, although more difficult, should be attainable by most patients.

GLYCEMIC CONTROL AND COMPLICATIONS: A SUMMARY OF EVIDENCE

Evidence relating hyperglycemia and/or other metabolic consequences of insulin deficiency to the development of vascular complications comes from older epidemiologic studies of European and North American patients with type 1 diabetes and from more recent controlled clinical trials from Scandinavia and North America. The Diabetes Control and Complications Trial (DCCT), sponsored by the National Institutes of Health, was a long-term prospective randomized controlled multicenter trial that studied the course of ~1,400 patients with type 1 diabetes. The patients were treated with intensive or conventional insulin regimens. The DCCT was designed to answer two questions: *1*) whether intensive glycemic control could prevent microvascular disease from developing and *2*) whether it could arrest or reverse early microvascular complications already present (with retinopathy as the primary endpoint). The study found that there is a link between glycemic control and development of diabetic complications. Intensively treated patients who achieve similar metabolic control can expect a 50–75% reduction in the risk of developing progression of retinopathy, nephropathy, and neuropathy after 8–9 yr. These changes begin to appear at 3–4 yr. Similar results have been reported in the smaller Stockholm Diabetes Intervention Study.

Prospective Clinical Trials

The DCCT examined whether intensive treatment with the goal of maintaining glucose concentrations close to the normal range could decrease the frequency and severity of diabetic complications. Investigators studied 1,441 patients with type 1 diabetes—726 with no retinopathy and 715 with mild retinopathy at baseline. Patients were randomly assigned to intensive therapy administered with insulin pumps or multiple injections of insulin guided by blood glucose monitoring or to conventional therapy with one or two insulin injections per day. The patients were followed a mean of 6.5 yr. Results showed that in the primary intervention cohort, intensive therapy reduced the mean risk of developing retinopathy by 76%. In the secondary intervention group, intensive therapy slowed the progression of retinopathy by 54% and reduced the development of proliferative retinopathy by 47%. In both groups combined, intensive therapy reduced the occurrence of microalbuminuria (>40 mg/24 h) by 39% and albuminuria (>300 mg/24 h) by 54%. Clinical neuropathy was reduced by 60%. The most important adverse effect was a threefold increase in severe hypoglycemia. Comparable results were seen in the Stockholm Diabetes Intervention Study after 5 and 8 yr.

After completion of the DCCT, most of the participants were enrolled in a long-term observational study titled the Epidemiology of Diabetes Interventions and Complications (EDIC). The difference in the median A1C values between the conventional therapy and intensive therapy groups during the 6.5 yr of the DCCT (average of 9.1% and 7.2%, respectively) narrowed during follow-up (median duration at 4 yr of 8.2% and 7.9%, respectively). Despite this small difference in glycemic control between the two groups at 4 yr of follow-up, the reduction in the risk of progressive retinopathy and nephropathy that resulted from intensive therapy persisted in EDIC. More recently, EDIC results at 6 yr of follow-up of these two groups showed a significant difference in the progression of the carotid intima-media thickness, a measure of atherosclerosis. These follow-up findings strongly support the implementation of intensive therapy as early as is safely possible and the maintenance of such therapy for as long as possible, with the expectation that a prolonged period of near-normal blood glucose levels will result in an even greater reduction in the risk of both microvascular and macrovascular complications in patients with type 1 diabetes.

Animal Studies

Strong experimental support for an association between metabolic abnormalities and vascular complications is found in animal studies. Animals that are rendered insulin deficient and hyperglycemic develop pathologic changes resembling early human retinopathy, nephropathy, and neuropathy. These changes can be prevented or ameliorated and, in some instances, even reversed by early intensive insulin treatment, by curing diabetes via pancreas or islet transplantation, or by transplanting the affected organ into a nondiabetic animal.

Other Causes of Diabetes

Microvascular disease also develops in some patients with diabetes resulting from removal or destruction of the islets caused by pancreatectomy, chronic pancreatitis, or toxicity (e.g., from the rodenticide Vacor). These observations further support the theory that loss of insulin secretion or some consequent metabolic derangement is responsible for microvascular abnormalities in patients with immune-mediated type 1 diabetes. Genetic predisposition may influence the development of microvascular, neuropathic, and other complications; however, hyperglycemia is a prerequisite to development of these complications.

Kidney Transplantation Observations

Normal kidneys transplanted into recipients with type 1 diabetes begin to show pathologic changes resembling diabetic nephropathy after several years. Normal kidneys transplanted into patients with successful whole-pancreas transplantation have less glomerulopathy than kidneys transplanted into patients treated with conventional therapy. These observations point to a causative role for the diabetic metabolic milieu.

Epidemiologic Studies

Several epidemiologic studies in patients with type 1 diabetes suggest that the higher the glucose level, the greater the incidence of microvascular disease.

GOALS OF TREATMENT

The physician and patient, with the diabetes management team and family, must set treatment goals together. If overlooked, this deceptively simple point often leads to failure. The physician convinced of the importance of targeted glycemic control in every case will be frustrated by a patient who does not understand the need for, or is unable to accept the goal or methods used to achieve, glycemic control. Conversely, the patient who wants blood glucose levels to be normal all the time and is truly willing to work for it will be frustrated by a physician who lacks the time, facilities, conviction, or training to help achieve this goal or who is unable to guide the patient to achieve a safe and realistic set of goals.

In addition to a clear agreement on goals, a good diabetes management team–patient treatment match requires open communication and appropriate patient education. At the tightest end of the treatment spectrum, the patient must have a sophisticated and practical understanding of physiology and pharmacology when striving to maintain normal glucose levels when, for example, exercising strenuously. In contrast, at the looser end, knowledge may be more rudimentary, but patients must at least know that to avoid diabetic ketoacidosis (DKA), they may have to take extra insulin on sick days when appetite is poor and common sense seems to dictate the reverse. Treatment must always be individualized with regard to specific goals. Goals should be realistic and achievable. Success in achieving small incremental steps is more likely to lead to a larger goal. Sometimes more can be gained by striving for less.

The physician and other team members should avoid seeming autocratic, moralistic, or judgmental. They should try to be understanding when goals are not met easily or quickly and should empathize with the patient's difficulty in paying daily attention to the never-ending demands of diabetes. It may help to work with the patient to identify obstacles to the treatment plan so the patient can address them. It is important to encourage the best goals achievable without demanding the impossible, unsafe, or impractical.

Setting individual patient glycemic targets should take into account the results of prospective randomized clinical trials, most notably the DCCT. This trial conclusively demonstrated that in patients with type 1 diabetes the risk of development or progression of retinopathy, nephropathy, and neuropathy is reduced 50–75% by intensive treatment regimens when compared with conventional treatment regimens. These benefits were observed with an average glycated hemoglobin (A1C) of 7.2% in intensively treated groups of patients compared with an A1C of 9.0% in conventionally treated groups of patients. The reduction in risk of these complications correlated continuously with the reduction in A1C produced by intensive treatment. This relationship implies that complete normalization of glycemic levels may prevent complications. The nondiabetic reference range for A1C in the DCCT was 4.0–6.0%. All nationally certified A1C measurements are now standardized to the DCCT assay range.

Self-monitoring of blood glucose (SMBG) targets in the DCCT were 70–120 mg/dl (3.9–6.7 mmol/l) before meals and at bedtime and <180 mg/dl (<10.0 mmol/l) when measured 1.5–2.0 h postprandially. However, these goals were associated with a threefold increased risk of severe hypoglycemia. Therefore, it may be appropriate to increase these targets (e.g., 90–130 mg/dl [5.0–7.2 mmol/l] before meals and 100–140 mg/dl [5.6–7.8 mmol/l] at bedtime) (Table 2.1). These targets should be further adjusted in patients with a history of recurrent severe hypoglycemia or hypoglycemia unawareness.

Individual treatment goals should take into account the patient's capacity to understand and carry out the treatment regimen, the patient's risk for severe hypoglycemia, and other patient factors that may increase risk or decrease benefit, e.g., very young or old age, end-stage renal disease, advanced cardiovascular or cerebrovascular disease, or other coexisting diseases that will materially shorten life expectancy.

The desired outcome of glycemic control in type 1 diabetes is to lower glycated hemoglobin (A1C or an equivalent measure of chronic glycemia) so as to achieve maximum prevention of complications with due regard for patient safety.

CLINICAL GOALS

Initial Goals

For the new-onset acutely decompensated patient or the previously diagnosed patient in poor control, goals should include

Table 2.1 Summary of Recommendations for Adults with Diabetes Mellitus

Glycemic control	
A1C	<7.0%*
Preprandial plasma glucose	90–130 mg/dl (5.0–7.2 mmol/l)
Peak postprandial plasma glucose	<180 mg/dl (<10.0 mmol/l)
Blood pressure	<130/80 mmHg
Lipids	
LDL	<100 mg/dl (<2.6 mmol/l)
Triglycerides†	<150 mg/dl (<1.7 mmol/l)
HDL	>40 mg/dl (>1.1 mmol/l)‡

From American Diabetes Association: Standards of medical care for patients with diabetes mellitus (Position Statement). *Diabetes Care* 26 (Suppl. 1):S33–S50, 2003.
*Referenced to a nondiabetic range of 4.0–6.0% using a DCCT-based assay.
†Current NCEP/ATP III guidelines suggest that in patients with triglycerides ≥200 mg/dl, the "non–HDL cholesterol" (total cholesterol minus HDL) be utilized. The goal is ≤130 mg/dl.
‡For women, it has been suggested that the HDL goal be increased by 10 mg/dl.

- eliminating ketosis
- returning to desirable body weight range by reversing water and extracellular electrolyte losses and replenishing lean body mass (protein and intracellular electrolytes)
- eliminating obvious consequences of hyperglycemia, e.g., gross polyuria and polydipsia, vaginitis or balanitis, recurrent infections, and visual blurring due to reversible refractive changes
- avoiding cerebral edema in cases of DKA

Additional Goals

Once the initial clinical goals have been achieved, additional goals should include

- near-normalization of blood glucose values and A1C with avoidance of severe hypoglycemia
- preventing symptoms of hyperglycemia, such as excessive thirst and urinary frequency, from disturbing sleep, school, work, social, or recreational activities
- preventing spontaneous and illness-induced ketosis
- maintaining weight within a desirable range
- stimulating catch-up growth and sexual maturation in children with poor glycemic control
- maintaining normal growth rate in children and adolescents
- maintaining maximum exercise tolerance and stamina
- maintaining a sense of psychosocial well-being and normal initiative in self-management

- minimizing self-treatable hypoglycemia and avoiding severe hypoglycemic seizures, accidents (e.g., while driving), and coma
- avoiding hospitalization
- for women, achieving normal fertility and pregnancy outcome
- sustaining normal family and marital relationships and sex life
- preventing diabetes-dictated or diabetes-oriented lifestyle (i.e., diabetes controlling the patient rather than vice versa)

In addition to the educational and clinical goals discussed above, patients and the diabetes management team should individualize glycemic control goals. It is desirable to aim for near-normalization of blood glucose, if this can be achieved without significant serious side effects (Table 2.2). All patients should be given the opportunity to pursue these goals using a flexible, individualized diabetes management program, based on an assessment of potential risks and benefits.

Assessors of Control

Diabetes control is assessed by the patient at home via SMBG and urine or blood ketones. At the office, longer-term glycemic control is assessed by results of glycohemoglobin tests. Many different types of glycohemoglobin assay methods are available to the routine clinical laboratory. Methods differ considerably with respect to the glycated components measured, interferences, and nondiabetic range. Glycated hemoglobin A_{1c} (A1C) has become the preferred standard for assessing glycemic control. As a result, the National Glycohemoglobin Standardization Program (NGSP) was formed in 1996 to standardize the A1C test to DCCT values. All manufacturers of A1C test assay methods are encouraged to seek NGSP certification on an annual basis, and all clinical laboratories are encouraged to do proficiency testing using whole-blood specimens. Generally, a 1% change in A1C levels corresponds to a change in mean blood glucose of 35 mg/dl (1.9 mmol/l). In nondiabetic individuals, A1C values are 4.0–6.0%.

The premeal SMBG goal for optimal treatment is similar to the 70–120 mg/dl (3.9–6.7 mmol/l) goal used in the DCCT. Over the course of that study, >75% of morning (fasting) glucose levels were >120 mg/dl (>6.7 mmol/l). In practice, most prebreakfast glucose levels will be between 80 and 160 mg/dl (4.4 and 8.9 mmol/l) in patients with A1C values <7.0% yet acceptable rates of severe hypoglycemia.

Table 2.2 Biochemical and Clinical Characteristics of Blood Glucose Near-Normalization

Optimal glycemic control (may be referred to as intensive) is characterized by	
■ A1C <7.0%	■ Peak postprandial SMBG <180 mg/dl (<10.0 mmol/l)
■ Preprandial SMBG 90–130 mg/dl (5.0–7.2 mmol/l)	■ Essentially no ketonuria
	■ Mean blood glucose levels 110–150 mg/dl (6.1–8.3 mmol/l)

In the past, when data compiled from diabetes specialty clinics in North America and Europe were analyzed, patients with type 1 diabetes have shown median A1C values of 8.0–9.0%. These correspond to mean blood glucose levels of ~200 mg/dl (~11.1 mmol/l). Adolescents with type 1 diabetes generally average 0.5–1.0% higher values and a blood glucose that is 20–40 mg/dl (1.1–2.2 mmol/l) higher than adults. Ninety-five percent of type 1 patients have an A1C of 5.0–13.0%. Levels as high as 20–25% are seen in the newly diagnosed and patients with very poor glycemic control.

Patients with hemoglobin variants (HbS, C, F) cannot have their glucose control measured with HbA_{1c} or HbA_1 assays using conventional high-performance liquid or cation-exchange chromatography. In these patients, glucose control can be assessed with radioimmunoassay methods for measuring HbA_{1c} and affinity chromatography methods for GHb.

Glycemic Control Goals

The following levels of glycemic control are appropriate for patients with type 1 diabetes.

- In all pregnant women and women attempting to conceive, seek "stringent" biochemical goals of intensive treatment (≤6.5% A1C, blood glucose 60–120 mg/dl [3.3–6.7 mmol/l]) by methods detailed below (see Pregnancy, page 146).
- In nonpregnant patients who are well informed about the risks and potential benefits of intensive insulin therapy and are motivated and suitably educable, seek an optimal level of control (<7.0% A1C). This is accomplished with average blood glucose levels of 110–150 mg/dl (6.1–8.3 mmol/l). These goals are sought if achievable without significant serious side effects. Day-to-day fluctuations in blood glucose level are unavoidable. If the patient does not sense or respond to hypoglycemia or has frequent severe hypoglycemia, goals should be set higher to reduce the risk of severe hypoglycemia.

Results of Optimal Control

At an optimal level of control, patients are entirely asymptomatic and may perceive a very good or excellent sense of well-being, energy, and exercise capacity and less disease-related anxiety compared with maintenance at poor control. They may also express a greater sense of control over the management of the disease if they use a flexible, individualized management program. However, they may experience increased mild self-treated and also severe hypoglycemic episodes. Some patients may feel excessively burdened by the required frequent monitoring, insulin administration methods, and constant dietary adherence. Negotiation (and renegotiation) of mutually acceptable goals will reduce the chances that patients will abandon reasonable self-care. In fact, treatment of type 1 diabetes always involves a negotiated therapeutic alliance between patient (and family) and the diabetes management team.

CONCLUSION

For patients with type 1 diabetes, the long-term benefits of optimal diabetes management appear extremely promising. A flexible, individualized diabetes management program utilizing the principles of intensive insulin therapy should be encouraged in almost all type 1 diabetes patients from onset. These benefits must be balanced in each patient against actual risks and costs. The diabetes management team together with the patient should set treatment goals on the basis of their own best judgment regarding individual patient capabilities and understanding.

BIBLIOGRAPHY

American Diabetes Association: Standards of medical care for patients with diabetes mellitus (Position Statement). *Diabetes Care* 26 (Suppl. 1):S33–S50, 2003

American Diabetes Association: Tests of glycemia with diabetes (Position Statement). *Diabetes Care* 26 (Suppl. 1):S106–S108, 2003

DCCT/EDIC Research Group: Intensive diabetes therapy and carotid intima-media thickness in type 1 diabetes. *N Engl J Med* 348:2294–2303, 2003

DCCT/EDIC Research Group: Retinopathy and nephropathy in patients with type 1 diabetes four years after a trial of intensive therapy. *N Engl J Med* 342:381–389, 2000

DCCT Research Group: The effect of intensive treatment of diabetes on the development and progression of long-term complications in insulin-dependent diabetes mellitus. *N Engl J Med* 329:977–986, 1993

DCCT Research Group: The relationship of glycemic exposure (HbA$_{1c}$) to the risk of development and progression of retinopathy in the Diabetes Control and Complications Trial. *Diabetes* 44:968–993, 1995

Klein R: Hyperglycemia and microvascular and macrovascular disease in diabetes. *Diabetes Care* 18:258–268, 1995

National Cholesterol Education Program (NCEP) Expert Panel on Detection, Evaluation, and Treatment of High Blood Cholesterol in Adults (Adult Treatment Panel III): Executive summary of the third report of the National Cholesterol Education Program (NCEP) Expert Panel on Detection, Evaluation, and Treatment of High Blood Cholesterol in Adults (Adult Treatment Panel III). *JAMA* 285:2486–2497, 2001

Pirart J: Diabetes mellitus and its degenerative complications: a prospective study of 4,400 patients observed between 1947 and 1973. *Diabetes Care* 1:168–188, 252–263, 1978

Reichard P, Nilsson BY, Rosenqvist U: The effect of long-term intensified insulin treatment on the development of microvascular complications of diabetes mellitus. *N Engl J Med* 329:304–309, 1993

Rohlfing CL, Wiedmeyer HM, Little RR, England JD, Tennill A, Goldstein DE: Defining the relationship between plasma glucose and HbA$_{1c}$: analysis of glucose profiles and HbA$_{1c}$ in the Diabetes Control and Complications Trial. *Diabetes Care* 25:275–278, 2002

Santiago JV: Lessons from the Diabetes Control and Complications Trial. *Diabetes* 42:1549–1554, 1993

Skyler JS: Tactics in type 1 diabetes. *Endocrinol Metab Clin North Am* 26:647–657, 1997

PATIENT SELF-MANAGEMENT EDUCATION

D iabetes management is a team effort. Physicians, nurses, dietitians, and other health care professionals contribute their expertise and long-term implementation to the design of therapeutic regimens that will enable patients to achieve the best possible metabolic control. The patient is at the center of the team and, supported by his or her family, has responsibility for day-to-day implementation of the treatment plan. In the case of children, the caregivers take on this responsibility. Therapy will be most effective if the patient understands the regimen, is not ambivalent about the value, and has mastered the skills to do required tasks correctly. Therefore, the clinical management of diabetes relies on patient self-management.

The importance of patient education is underscored by the DCCT, which demonstrated that intensive treatment of diabetes, with great demands in patient self-management, can prevent or delay the long-term complications of diabetes. Intensive therapy brings an increased risk of hypoglycemia, making patient education critical in providing safety. This section provides an overview of diabetes patient education, including information on the principles, process, content, and guidelines for incorporating education into clinical practice. Currently, several terms, including diabetes self-management education and diabetes self-management training, are being used to describe patient education in diabetes. They will be used interchangeably in this manual. However, for reimbursement purposes, diabetes self-management training is the preferred terminology.

GENERAL PRINCIPLES

The goal of diabetes self-management education is to provide patients with the knowledge, skills, and motivation to incorporate diabetes self-management into their daily life. To meet this goal, diabetes education must include teaching patients the new information they need to know about diabetes management, training them in the various skills they need for treatment procedures, assisting them in devising methods to fit the regimen into their lifestyle, and helping them reconcile diabetes care with their quality of life so they are motivated to manage their disease.

Ideally, a diabetes management team should be involved in patient education. Many physicians may not have a diabetes education team available in their practice setting and need to refer patients, if possible, to a diabetes education program or to diabetes educators. Physicians can develop a team approach by collaborating with diabetes educators working in diabetes education programs or in private practice. The national office of the American Association of Diabetes Educators can provide names of certified diabetes educators. Also, the American Diabetes Association's Education Recognition Program has identified diabetes education programs that meet the National Standards for Diabetes Self-Management Education. This list is available on the Association's web site at www.diabetes.org/recognition/education.

Diabetes self-management education is a planned process that requires time, materials, space, and professional expertise (Table 2.3). The knowledge and skills patients need to implement their treatment regimen cannot be acquired during

Table 2.3 Process of Diabetes Self-Management Education

Assessment	Identify patient's individual education needs
Planning	Set goals for education based on the assessment and select teaching/learning strategies
Implementation	Provide the planned education in an environment that supports learning
Documentation	Document educational activities to inform other members of the diabetes management team and to record the care provided
Evaluation	Measure the impact of education by testing knowledge and skills and by evaluating behavioral and metabolic outcomes

a quick interaction on the day of diagnosis or in a single instructional session in a physician's office. Moreover, patient education is an ongoing component of diabetes care, not a one-time referral.

For the newly diagnosed patient, a staged approach to education should be used, with the initial teaching focused on the critical information that will enable the individual, or caregiver, to implement the regimen at home (Table 2.4). Once the patient is comfortable with the fundamental components of the regimen, teaching can be expanded to provide more in-depth information and to introduce

Table 2.4 Basic Education at Diagnosis: Survival Skills

Topics and the critical knowledge and skills patients need to manage their diabetes at home include:

General facts	Explain the need for daily insulin injections and that treatment of diabetes involves insulin, diet, exercise, and SMBG
Medications	Measure insulin dosage accurately, inject correctly, and understand timing of injections and how to handle insulin and supplies
Nutrition	Explain the relationship of food, insulin, and blood glucose, and the amount, type of food, and times to eat to maximize blood glucose control
Exercise	Explain the relationships of exercise, food, and insulin and how to prevent hypoglycemia from exercise
Monitoring	Perform accurate SMBG and urine or blood ketone tests
Hyperglycemia and hypoglycemia	Differentiate the signs and symptoms of high and low blood glucose levels and know what actions to take for each situation; know when to seek immediate medical assistance for intercurrent illness, hyperglycemia, or ketonuria
Use of the health care system	Identify how to obtain insulin supplies, whom to call for professional advice, and how to get help in an emergency

additional topics. Continuing education across the life span provides opportunities for learning new management techniques and for making adjustments in the regimen to accommodate lifestyle changes, growth, and aging.

To be effective, diabetes self-management education must be individualized. Teaching methods, however, need not be limited to individual instruction. Group classes and self-study methods can supplement individual instruction and offer advantages in meeting different learning styles and in efficient use of teaching time. Information from all sources must be consistent, whether provided by different health professionals or from diverse instructional materials. Therefore, all members of the diabetes management team need to be aware of the content of the education program.

SELF-MANAGEMENT EDUCATION PROCESS

Diabetes self-management education is a systematic procedure that starts with an assessment of individual educational needs to guide planning of teaching/learning strategies, followed by implementation of the plan and documentation of the process, and concluding with evaluation of health outcomes. Although terms may be different, the process mimics the traditional steps clinicians use to diagnose and treat patients. Understanding the commonalties of patient education and medical care facilitates integration of education into the clinical management of diabetes.

Assessment

The first step in the educational process is an assessment to provide physical, psychosocial, and educability data to determine an individual education plan. Information obtained in this assessment can guide both treatment and education decisions. For example, if assessment shows that the individual has limited learning skills, treatment with a simple insulin regimen versus a complex algorithm of dose adjustments would be appropriate, with educational strategies providing pictorial instruction materials, demonstration with return demonstration, and a plan for evaluating accurate performance at home.

The education assessment also focuses on the three key areas of the learning process: cognitive/knowledge, psychomotor/skills, and affective/attitude. To develop teaching strategies, the educator needs to evaluate each patient to determine specific knowledge that needs to be acquired; skills that need to be mastered; and personal attitudes toward diabetes, health care, and life that will influence that patient's diabetes self-management.

As a general framework, the educational assessment should include

- demographic information: age, gender, level of education, occupation, and family status
- medical history: height; weight; blood pressure; blood glucose values (A1C, fasting, plasma glucose, and self-monitoring results); blood lipid values; medications (prescribed and over-the-counter); allergies; other medical problems; general health status, including smoking, alcohol

consumption, sexual activity, and use of social drugs; and health service or
resource utilization
- diabetes history: type of diabetes; duration of diabetes; current treatment
plan, including medication, diet, exercise, monitoring, and problems with
adherence; acute and chronic complications; family history; and previous
diabetes education
- dietary habits: meal times and locations, snacking patterns, food preferences, resources for food preparation, and previous diet instructions
(note that medical nutrition therapy includes a more detailed history; see
Nutrition, page 85)
- physical activity: work/school activity, recreational activity
- social history: information on household, extended family, social network,
cultural factors, religious practices, health beliefs, and current health
practices
- economic profile: income, insurance, transportation resources, and neigh-
borhood environment
- lifestyle: activities of daily living, including work, school, and leisure time;
for children, information on after-school, weekend, and summer activities
- psychosocial status: feelings about diabetes, personal relationships (with
spouse, partner, parents, family, peers), developmental stages in life-cycle,
history of sleep or eating disorders, stress, anxiety, or depression; health
goals
- education factors: literacy, computational skills, readiness to learn, preferred learning methods, visual acuity, hearing loss, and dexterity
- knowledge and skill level in each of the 10 content areas of the National
Standards for Diabetes Self-Management Education

Additional information will be required to develop educational plans to meet
the idiosyncratic needs of individual patients. Also, as with nutrition, each member of the diabetes management team will use a more extensive assessment
specific to their area of expertise.

Planning Educational Strategies

The assessment identifies the topics that need to be included in the education plan and teaching methods that would be most effective. From this analysis,
educational goals are developed for each patient. The educational goals must correspond with therapeutic goals established by the diabetes management team
and diabetes management goals set by the patient. If the diabetes management
team is focused on normalization of blood glucose and the patient is focused on
making a minimum number of lifestyle changes, teaching will not be effective
until there is agreement. Once goals are established, measurable behavioral objectives are developed with the patient to clearly identify steps that will be used to
achieve these goals.

The education plan delineates what is to be taught when, how, where, and by
whom. There are numerous teaching strategies that can be used with a patient
(Table 2.5). For a newly diagnosed patient, the plan would specify topics that need

Table 2.5 Teaching Strategies

Methods

- Individual instruction: education can be tailored to individual learning needs and focused on specific details of patient's self-management plan
- Group classes: efficient use of educator time, patients benefit from social support and peer learning
- Self-study: flexible, allows patient to pace learning, educator should monitor and evaluate progress

Techniques

- Short lecture: effective for presenting new information
- Discussion: allows patient to personalize information, ask questions, disclose feelings, and share experiences
- Skills training: provides "hands on" learning; educator demonstrates, patient practices then performs a return demonstration and receives feedback from educator
- Problem solving: allows patients to integrate information on several topics, such as diet, insulin, and exercise, and to test their knowledge in hypothetical situations
- Role playing: can be used to reinforce learning (patient plays educator role), to practice social skills (explaining diabetes to friends), and to explore personal problems (family stress)
- Case studies: provide an objective approach to learning that can be used for planning, problem solving, and to help patients identify errors they are making in their diabetes self-management
- Self-assessment: blood glucose records, food diaries, and exercise logs can be used to help patients recognize problems in their diabetes self-management and often to identify solutions

Materials

- Printed materials: can be used to reinforce teaching, for self-study, and as an information resource for future needs (e.g., sick-day guidelines)
- Audio and visual aides: slides, films, overheads, audiotapes and videotapes, food models and labels, sample diabetes products, and dolls and puppets are effective in enhancing learning
- Interactive learning programs: available in printed, audio, visual, and computer formats; allow individuals to learn at their own pace, with frequent evaluation to provide feedback on learning
- Games: crossword puzzles, board games, and group games introduce fun into the educational process while enhancing participant learning
- Group classes on balancing the insulin–diet–exercise triad and on preventing and treating hypoglycemia
- A case study with questions to evaluate learning and problem-solving skills

to be covered immediately to provide the patient with the "survival skills" necessary to manage his or her diabetes at home (Table 2.4). Teaching methods could include

- one-on-one sessions with the dietitian to develop a meal plan
- one-on-one sessions with the diabetes educator to learn insulin injection and monitoring techniques

- observation of patient injection and monitoring skills by staff nurses
- a videotape describing pathophysiology

The plan would include methods for evaluating learning accomplished in the initial phase, steps to reinforce what has been taught, and resources for obtaining in-depth education within a reasonable time frame.

Implementation

Teaching can take place in a classroom, at bedside, in an office, in the home, in the cafeteria, or in a number of other settings. Whatever space is used, it is critical that the environment support learning and reinforce the importance of the educational process. There should be adequate lighting and furnishings and minimal distractions. Education sessions should be scheduled at specific times. Scheduling will help ensure that teaching takes place; deter the potential for tests, visitors, or other situations receiving priority; and establish the concept that education is a specific part of diabetes care. The same measures used to reinforce routine clinical appointments should be used, including written information giving the appointment time, location (with directions if needed), and the name(s) and telephone number(s) of the educator(s).

Documentation

Documentation of education is as important as documentation of treatment procedures. Documentation provides a means of communication among the diabetes management team as well as substantiating the provision of educational care. Documentation can be included in progress notes in the patient's medical chart, maintained in education charts, or written in correspondence and reports. Whatever method of documentation is used, a permanent record of a patient's educational experience must be maintained.

Evaluation

The effectiveness of the educational plan is evaluated in several ways. First, assessment will provide measures of knowledge gained, skills acquired, and changes in attitudes. This type of evaluation often is included in the implementation process to allow for reinforcement in areas where the patient exhibits weaknesses. Periodic assessment will provide measures of lapses in knowledge, skills, or attitudes that can be remedied with a refresher course. Another evaluation procedure measures changes in behavior. This evaluation takes place some time after education (1–3 mo) to measure whether the behavior is being maintained. The behavioral objectives developed during the planning phase may be used, or a different set of objectives can be set at the completion of education as an outgrowth of the learning process. A third approach evaluates the effectiveness of education by examining treatment goals, such as lower A1C, minimal hypoglycemia, or absence of ketoacidosis. All forms of evaluation yield an assessment of additional educational needs of the patient.

CONTENT OF DIABETES SELF-MANAGEMENT EDUCATION

Topics to be included in diabetes patient education are numerous and vary according to type of diabetes, patient age, and other individual characteristics. The National Standards for Diabetes Self-Management Education specify that programs should be able to provide information in 10 content areas. The suggested topics are listed below with basic teaching points for type 1 diabetes:

- **Diabetes disease process and treatments.** Type 1 diabetes is a chronic metabolic disorder in which the body no longer produces insulin required to use food for energy. Lack of insulin can be life threatening. Daily insulin injections are essential and need to be balanced with meals and physical activity to manage diabetes. Understanding the interactions among the three and their impact on blood glucose levels is important in making self-management decisions. Self-monitoring values provide information that can be used to make adjustments in one or more of the three therapeutic agents.
- **Nutrition.** Food is an important part of diabetes treatment and health. The amount, type, and timing of meals and snacks must be balanced with insulin and exercise to maintain good blood glucose control. Meal plans should be individualized to reflect food preferences and daily schedules, provide optimum nutrition, and make diabetes self-management as effective as possible.
- **Physical activity.** Physical activity is recommended for health and diabetes management. Physical activity can affect blood glucose levels, usually by lowering them. Planning can prevent hypoglycemia that may occur during or after exercise.
- **Medications.** Insulin must be taken daily as prescribed. It is important to know the type and amount of insulin to be taken and times to administer insulin and to understand the action and duration of the prescribed insulin. Correct techniques for drawing up and injecting insulin are critical to ensure that the dose is accurate. Glucagon is used to treat severe hypoglycemia. Family members and close friends need to know how to administer glucagon.
- **Monitoring and use of results.** Proper technique is crucial to achieve reliable results. Blood glucose monitoring results can be used to assess the effectiveness of the treatment regimen, identify low blood glucose levels requiring treatment to prevent hypoglycemia, indicate high blood glucose levels possibly associated with illness, show the effect of different meals and activities on blood glucose, and guide decisions on when to call health care providers. Urine or blood testing for ketones is required during times of physical or emotional stress.
- **Prevention, detection, and treatment of acute complications (hypoglycemia, hyperglycemia, and illness).** Hypoglycemia comes on quickly. Therefore, it is important to recognize the signs and symptoms of hypoglycemia and to know how to prevent and treat it (Table 2.6). Hyperglycemia that cannot be explained by diet or another aspect of the regimen (e.g., decrease in exercise or inadequate insulin delivery or amount) may indicate illness. Patients with type 1 diabetes can develop

Table 2.6 Sample Patient Guidelines for Treating Mild Hypoglycemia: 15/15 Rule

If blood glucose falls below 70 mg/dl:

- Eat 15 g carbohydrate, preferably in the form of glucose products
- Wait 15 min—retest, and if blood glucose remains <70 mg/dl, treat with another 15 g carbohydrate
- Repeat testing and treating until blood glucose returns to normal range
- If >1 h to next meal, add additional 15 g carbohydrate to maintain blood glucose in normal range

Sources of carbohydrate

Glucose products (preferred):

Glucose tablets	4–5 g/tablet
Glutose gel	15 g/dose
Insta-glucose gel	24 g tube/one-dose tube

Food/beverages (use if above not available), 15-g portions:

Graham crackers	3
Saltine crackers	6
Raisins	2 Tbsp
Syrup or honey	1 Tbsp
Juice (apple/orange)	1/2 cup
Soft drink (regular)	1/2 cup
Skim milk	1 cup
Ginger ale	3/4 cup

Note: Severe hypoglycemia needs to be treated by someone knowledgeable about diabetes. Guidelines should be available in schools and work sites. If the patient cannot swallow well, glucagon must be used instead of oral treatment.

DKA when ill. Therefore, guidelines for sick days need to be followed carefully (Table 2.7). Family members, friends, coworkers, and teachers need to know how to respond in case of emergencies.

- **Prevention, detection, treatment, and rehabilitation of chronic complications.** Chronic complications are a serious concern in diabetes. Steps that can reduce the risk of complications include maintaining blood glucose levels as near to normal as feasible, not smoking, having annual eye exams, controlling blood pressure and blood lipid levels, and taking preventive care of feet.
- **Behavior change strategies, goal setting, risk factor reduction, and problem solving.** Most aspects of diabetes management require changes in behavior. Behavior change is not simply willpower. Techniques such as goal setting, contracting, and problem solving are helpful in changing habits to reduce health risks and improve diabetes control. Attention should be addressed to risk factors for diabetic complications, including cardiovascular disease. Achieving optimal glucose control may deter the complications of diabetes. However, tight control brings an increased risk

Table 2.7 Sample Patient Guidelines for Sick-Day Management

Illness can make diabetes more difficult to manage. Even when you do not feel well, you must take your insulin, test blood glucose and urine or blood ketones, drink fluids, and eat some food. You will need ketone strips and food such as regular gelatin and soft drinks. Therefore, planning ahead for sick days is important. The following guidelines will help you during mild illnesses.

Monitoring

Blood glucose and urine (or blood) ketones need to be tested frequently during illness, often every 2–4 h. Test for ketones if you have unexplainable blood glucose values >250 mg/dl or if you feel ill, even if blood glucose values are normal. Write down the values and call a member of your diabetes management team when premeal blood glucose values stay >250 mg/dl and/or when you measure moderate or large ketones.

Insulin

Never stop taking insulin even if vomiting and unable to eat. Your body often needs more insulin during illness. Therefore, your health care professional may ask you to take supplemental insulin (a correction bolus) according to results of blood glucose monitoring.

Food and fluid intake

Use small meals and eat more frequently when you are ill. Soft foods or liquids are often tolerated best. Eating about 10–15 g carbohydrate every 1–2 h is usually sufficient. Foods and beverages containing about 15 g carbohydrate include

1/2 cup regular gelatin	3/4 cup regular ginger ale
1/2 cup vanilla ice cream	1/2 cup regular soft drink
1/2 cup custard	1/2 cup orange or apple juice
1 regular double Popsicle	1 cup Gatorade
1/2 cup applesauce	1 cup creamed soup

Fluid intake is essential during illness. If vomiting, diarrhea, or fever is present, take small quantities of liquids every 15–30 min. Clear broth, tea, and other fluids can supplement liquids containing carbohydrate.

Seek medical attention when you have

- Fever >100°F
- Persistent diarrhea
- Vomiting and are unable to take fluids for >4 h
- Blood glucose levels that are difficult to control with or without ketones (see information above on monitoring)

- Severe abdominal pain
- Other unexplained symptoms
- Illness that persists over 24 h

Physician's # —————————————— Pharmacy # ——————————————

---

of hypoglycemia. Individuals with diabetes need to be responsible for their diabetes management, which includes working with their diabetes management team to select the treatment plan that meets their personal goals for health.

- **Psychosocial adjustment.** Fear, anger, and denial are common responses to the diagnosis of diabetes. The day-by-day demands of diabetes management can be frustrating. Stress may cause problems with blood glucose control. Coping skills, stress reduction techniques, and professional counseling can help the patient handle the psychosocial impact of diabetes. Type 1 diabetes affects the whole family. Family members, friends, co-workers, and teachers need to know about diabetes and how to support the regimen.

- **Preconception care and pregnancy.** Optimal glucose control will reduce risks to the infant in pregnancies complicated by diabetes. Women with type 1 diabetes need to achieve excellent blood glucose control before becoming pregnant (optimally for 3 mo before conception). Tight blood glucose control needs to be maintained throughout pregnancy.

ADDITIONAL TOPICS OF IMPORTANCE FOR TYPE 1 DIABETES

- **Use of health care system and community resources.** People with diabetes need to be good consumers of the health care system and of community resources. Ongoing versus episodic care is important. Telephone numbers of diabetes management team members and emergency services should be readily available for use by family and friends as well as the individual with diabetes. Identifying resources in the community for supplies, services, information, and support groups makes day-to-day diabetes management easier.
- **Patient identification.** Wearing an identification bracelet or necklace at all times is strongly encouraged so that diabetes can be identified if severe hypoglycemia or an accident occurs.
- **Driving a motor vehicle.** Special care should be taken to prevent hypoglycemia while driving a car, truck, motorboat, or any other powered vehicle. Blood glucose levels should be checked before driving especially if the last meal was more than 3 h earlier or if the trip will be long, and low blood glucose values should be treated appropriately (Table 2.6). Supplies for SMBG and treating hypoglycemia should be carried in the vehicle at all times. If symptoms of hypoglycemia occur, driving should stop immediately and not be resumed until blood glucose levels are in the normal range for at least 10 min.
- **Travel guidelines.** Insulin and diabetes supplies sufficient for the entire trip need to be carried with the traveler and not put into checked baggage. Food to treat hypoglycemia and for a meal that may be delayed by late arrival should be carried as well. Prescriptions for insulin and syringes should be taken along as well, in case the need to purchase supplies does occur.
- **Career guidance.** Jobs that have erratic schedules, have long periods between meals, lack the flexibility to stop work and test blood glucose levels, or have other conditions make diabetes management more challenging. The Americans with Disabilities Act requires employers to make reasonable accommodations for employees with disabilities, including diabetes. The person with diabetes along with his or her supervisor and diabetes management team can identify ways to modify a job to accommodate the demands of work plus diabetes management.

- **Orientation and continuing education for school personnel.** Parents and the diabetes management team will want to work together to create a safe and supportive environment for school-age children.

INCORPORATING PATIENT EDUCATION IN CLINICAL PRACTICE

Patient education is essential for management of type 1 diabetes. However, all medical practice settings are not equipped to provide diabetes self-management training. Moreover, the complexity of type 1 diabetes, particularly when treated with intensive therapy, requires health care providers to have special expertise in diabetes. Physicians who specialize in the treatment of diabetes and who see many patients with type 1 diabetes can develop a team relationship with diabetes educators in the community, if hiring educators on a full- or part-time basis is not feasible. Systems such as health maintenance organizations, preferred provider organizations, and affiliations with hospitals offer potential resources for diabetes educators that can work with a number of physicians to maximize the economy of this specialized type of care. Physicians practicing in an area where there are education programs that have achieved American Diabetes Association Recognition may refer patients to programs that meet the National Standards. The local American Diabetes Association office maintains a list of recognized programs in their area. This list is also available on the Association's web site (www. diabetes.org/recognition/education).

To establish a team approach to diabetes self-management education, health professionals should *1*) share a common philosophy toward diabetes management and *2*) develop efficient methods for communicating about patient care and education to ensure that a consistent message is given to the patient. Forms can be helpful in documenting the educational process in a concise format that allows team members to keep abreast of each others' activities and to reinforce all areas of education. Communication by fax and computers offers the opportunity for expedient transfer of information among health professionals not working in the same location. Forms, if placed in the front of a chart or a similar place routinely used in providing patient care, can serve as a prompt to educate while providing routine medical care.

Diabetes education materials can be obtained from the American Diabetes Association, from companies manufacturing pharmaceuticals and diabetes equipment and supplies, and through a number of additional resources available through the National Diabetes Information Clearinghouse (www.NIDDK.NIH. gov).

CONCLUSION

Patients with type 1 diabetes need self-management education to be able to implement their treatment regimen. Education should be individualized to reflect the diabetes treatment regimen and learning characteristics of each patient. Self-management training is a systematic patient care process that requires educators with expertise in diabetes and resources in time and materials. Physicians should use a team approach to manage individuals with type 1 diabetes with self-management education integrated into the clinical care of the patient.

BIBLIOGRAPHY

American Association of Diabetes Educators: *A CORE Curriculum for Diabetes Educators.* 5th ed. Chicago, IL, American Association of Diabetes Educators, 2003

American Diabetes Association: *Diabetes Education Goals.* Alexandria, VA, American Diabetes Association, 2002

American Diabetes Association: *Life with Diabetes: A Series of Teaching Outlines by the Michigan Diabetes Research and Training Center.* 2nd ed. Alexandria, VA, American Diabetes Association, 2000

American Diabetes Association: Standards of medical care for patients with diabetes mellitus (Position Statement). *Diabetes Care* 26 (Suppl. 1):S33–S50, 2003

American Diabetes Association: National Standards for Diabetes Self-Management Education. *Diabetes Care* 26 (Suppl. 1):S149–S156, 2003

Anderson BJ, Rubin RR (Eds.): *Practical Psychology for Diabetes Clinicians.* 2nd ed. Alexandria, VA, American Diabetes Association, 2002

Anderson RM, Funnell MM, Burkhart N, Gillard ML, Nwankwo R: *101 Tips for Behavior Change in Diabetes Education.* Alexandria, VA, American Diabetes Association, 2002

Funnell MM, Anderson RM, Burkhart N, Gillard ML, Nwankwo R: *101 Tips for Diabetes Self-Management Education.* Alexandria, VA, American Diabetes Association, 2002

Kanzer-Lewis G: *Patient Education: You Can Do It!* Alexandria, VA, American Diabetes Association, 2003

Michigan Diabetes Research and Training Center: *Teenagers with Type 1 Diabetes: A Curriculum for Adolescents and Families.* Alexandria, VA, American Diabetes Association, 2001

Tools of Therapy

Exercise

Highlights
Tools of Therapy

INSULIN TREATMENT

■ Patients with type 1 diabetes are dependent on insulin to survive.

■ Ninety-eight percent of the insulin prescribed is made chemically identical to human insulin by recombinant DNA technology; 2% of the insulin prescribed is of animal origin obtained from pork pancreas.

■ Insulin analogs have been developed by modifying the amino acid sequence of the human insulin molecule. Insulin preparations are classified by duration of action (rapid, short, intermediate, and long acting) (Table 3.1).

■ The insulin regimen should be tailored to the needs of the individual patient. Therapy adjustments should be based on actual glycemic values obtained from patient self-monitoring of blood glucose (SMBG) rather than on "textbook" predictions of insulin action.

■ It is nearly impossible to adequately treat type 1 diabetes with once-daily insulin. Twice-daily insulin injections consist of the "split and mixed" combination of short- (or rapid-) and intermediate-acting insulin before breakfast and before supper. Generally, it is not possible to achieve near-normal glycemic levels with two injections per day.

■ More physiological multiple-component "flexible" regimens emphasize the difference between basal and prandial (bolus) insulin. These insulin regimens consist of

- three or more daily injections (prandial/bolus and basal insulins)
- insulin pump therapy

■ Insulin needs may fluctuate during the first weeks or months of treatment. If a honeymoon phase occurs, insulin dose must be appropriately reduced, occasionally to as little as 0.1–0.3 units/kg/day, but it should not be discontinued or replaced with an oral hypoglycemic agent.

■ Instructions for intensifying insulin therapy are found in Table 3.4. Continuous subcutaneous insulin infusion is an alternative that offers advantages in lifestyle flexibility and glycemic control.

■ Regimens using insulin algorithms place more demands on both patient and physician than does a fixed course of treatment, but they provide greater flexibility in lifestyle. All forms of intensive therapy require high degrees of long-term commitment and flexibility on the part of the patient, the family, and the diabetes management team.

■ Common problems associated with insulin therapy are detailed in Common Problems in Long-Term Therapy.

MONITORING

■ Patients can only manage their diabetes effectively and safely if they self-monitor. This includes self-monitoring of blood glucose as well as urine or blood ketone monitoring as needed and careful record-keeping.

■ Monitoring allows objective goals for therapy and a means to measure the efficacy of changes in therapy.

■ SMBG is the established monitoring method that allows

• detection and prevention of hypoglycemia and hyperglycemia
• adjustment of insulin, diet, and physical activity to achieve target blood glucose levels

■ Four SMBG measurements every day—before breakfast, lunch, supper, and bedtime—usually provide the necessary information sufficient to adjust insulin and diet. Additional tests are needed in the middle of the night to minimize the occurrence of nocturnal hypoglycemia, as well as when exercising, on sick days, or when a schedule has changed. Postprandial monitoring (1–2 h after the start of the meal) is helpful when pregnant or when glycemic goals have not been achieved with premeal glucose testing (Table 3.6).

■ Continuous or intermittent glucose monitoring of interstitial fluid is available to provide additional information to adjust insulin, exercise, and diet to optimize glycemic control and prevent hypoglycemia

■ A properly performed A1C provides the best available index of chronic glucose levels and is highly reliable.

NUTRITION

■ The overall goal of medical nutrition therapy (MNT) for type 1 diabetes is to enable patients to attain blood glucose levels as near normal as possible by integrating exogenous insulin into their usual eating and activity patterns. The MNT prescription should be individualized based on nutrition assessment and treatment goals. In general, recommendations follow nutrition guidelines for the general population:

• Calorie levels should be prescribed to achieve and maintain reasonable body weight.

- Protein intakes of 10–20% of calories are adequate to support health; intakes of ≤0.8 g/kg/day (~10% daily calories) are recommended for individuals showing evidence of diabetic nephropathy.
- Fat consumption should be moderate, with saturated fat limited to <10% of calories.
- Carbohydrate foods, such as grains, vegetables, and fruits, are rich sources of vitamins, minerals, and dietary fiber, and a liberal intake is encouraged. Sugars differ from starches in nutrient content but not in glycemic effect. For type 1 diabetes, the total amount of carbohydrate in a meal, rather than the source, should guide estimation of insulin dosage.
- Vitamin and mineral requirements of individuals with diabetes are the same as the general population. Supplementation is advised if conditions create a deficiency.

■ Insulin therapy regimens using multiple daily doses of insulin allows greater flexibility in eating patterns than does conventional therapy. Blood glucose levels obtained by self-monitoring can be used to make adjustments in diet and insulin regimen to maximize blood glucose control.

■ The complexity of integrating nutrition and insulin therapies and the importance of diabetes self-management education require a coordinated team approach to care for individuals with type 1 diabetes.

■ MNT for diabetes is based on an assessment of the individual's metabolic and lifestyle parameters, implemented through a nutrition self-management plan and evaluated through nutrition-related outcomes such as blood glucose and lipid levels. Patients and their families should be actively involved in setting nutrition goals, developing the self-management plan, and evaluating treatment effectiveness through SMBG levels.

■ Registered dietitians have the expertise to design the nutrition intervention and to counsel patients on nutrition self-management. Nutritional counseling for newly diagnosed patients with type 1 diabetes should be provided in stages to allow the patient time to adjust to the treatment regimen. Nutritional care cannot be limited to diagnosis but must continue throughout the patient's life span. Follow-up may be appropriate every 3–6 mo for children and every 6–12 mo for adults.

EXERCISE

■ Exercise should be an integral part of the treatment plan for patients with type 1 diabetes.

■ Physiological responses to exercise in nondiabetic people and in patients with type 1 diabetes are described in Table 3.13. For the type 1 diabetes patient, plasma insulin levels during and after exercise are critical determinants of response.

■ Potential benefits of exercise are explained on pages 109–110. Regular exercise improves cardiovascular risk factors and may

- aid in weight control
- heighten sense of well-being

■ Potential risks of exercise include destabilization of metabolic control, e.g.,

- hypoglycemia during or after exercise (most likely with sporadic exercise)
- hyperglycemia to the point of ketoacidosis (if diabetes is uncontrolled or ketones are present before beginning activity)

■ A preexercise medical evaluation should be performed regardless of the patient's age.

■ Exercise should be prescribed with caution in patients with

- unstable blood glucose values
- cardiovascular disease, neuropathy that results in loss of sensation, or proliferative retinopathy
- hypoglycemia unawareness

■ Guidelines for safe exercise are addressed in Table 3.15. They include

- monitoring blood glucose and taking appropriate action
- altering food or insulin if needed
- carrying short-acting carbohydrate and identification
- monitoring intensity of exercise
- avoiding trauma to joints, muscle, or ligaments as well as to the skin of the feet

Tools of Therapy

INSULIN TREATMENT

Type 1 diabetes mellitus is characterized by a near-absolute deficiency in endogenous insulin secretion within days or months after initial diagnosis. Affected patients are dependent on exogenous insulin to survive for the duration of their lives. Insulin injections are the mainstay of treatment and must be individualized for each patient.

INSULIN PREPARATIONS

Insulin is obtained from pork pancreas or is made chemically identical to human insulin by recombinant DNA technology. Insulin analogs have been developed by modifying the amino acid sequence of the human insulin molecule. Insulin preparations are generally classified by duration of action (rapid, short, intermediate, and long acting). Many insulin preparations are available; as a practical matter, health professionals should familiarize themselves with several of them and learn to use them rationally (Tables 3.1 and 3.2).

Species and Purity

In the United States today, at least 98% of insulin used is human insulin, prepared by recombinant DNA techniques. Also produced by recombinant DNA technology are insulin analogs. Two rapid-onset, short-duration analogs (insulin lispro and insulin aspart) and one long-acting analog (insulin glargine) are available, and other analogs are in development (see chapter on Emerging Therapies). Two insulins (NPH and regular) are of pork origin marketed under the trade name Iletin II by Lilly. All insulin preparations sold in the United States are highly purified and contain less than one part per million of impurities. Such purification is associated with a reduced incidence of insulin antibodies, less insulin allergy, and less lipoatrophy at the injection site than previous less purified preparations. Nevertheless, like all foreign proteins, animal insulins are antigenic. Pork insulin differs from the human molecule by two amino acids. Human insulin is the least antigenic insulin available.

The clinician should be aware that human insulin may act quicker, peak earlier, and last a shorter time than animal insulins. Lipoatrophy at the injection site, probably related to impurities, has become uncommon with either human or pure pork preparations.

Duration of Action

Although insulins are classified into rapid-, short-, intermediate-, and long-acting preparations, actual insulin effects do not always coincide with such simple descriptions. For example, local subcutaneous tissue conditions not clearly

Table 3.1 Insulins Sold in the United States

Product	Manufacturer	Strength
Rapid-acting (onset <15 min; usual duration 3–5 h)		
Human analog		
Humalog (insulin lispro)*†	Lilly	U-100
NovoLog (insulin aspart)*†	Novo Nordisk	U-100
Short-acting (usual onset 0.5–1.0 h; usual duration 3–6 h)		
Human		
Humulin R (regular)*	Lilly	U-100
Novolin R (regular)*†	Novo Nordisk	U-100
Human Buffered Regular (Velosulin)	Novo Nordisk	U-100
Pork		
Iletin II R (regular)	Lilly	U-100, U-500
Intermediate-acting (usual onset 3–6 h; usual duration 12–20 h)		
Human		
Humulin L (lente)	Lilly	U-100
Humulin N (NPH)*	Lilly	U-100
Novolin N (NPH)*†	Novo Nordisk	U-100
Pork		
Iletin II N (NPH)	Lilly	U-100
Long-acting (usual onset 4–6 h; usual duration 18–24 h)		
Human		
Humulin U (ultralente)	Lilly	U-100
Human Analog		
Lantus (insulin glargine)	Aventis	U-100
Premixed combinations		
Human		
Humulin 50/50 (50% NPH, 50% regular)	Lilly	U-100
Humulin 70/30 (70% NPH, 30% regular)*	Lilly	U-100
Novolin 70/30 (70% NPH, 30% regular)*†	Novo Nordisk	U-100
Human Analog		
Humalog 75/25 (75% NPL, 25% lispro)*†	Lilly	U-100
NovoLog 70/30 (70% NPA, 30% aspart)*†	Novo Nordisk	U-100

*Indicates availability in cartridges for pens, in addition to vials. †Indicates availability in "prefilled" disposable pens, in addition to cartridges and vials.

Table 3.2 Insulins by Comparative Action

	Onset (h)	Peak (h)	Effective duration (h)
Rapid acting			
Insulin lispro (analog)*	0.25–0.5	0.5–2.5	≤5
Insulin aspart (analog)*	<0.20	1–3	3–5
Short acting			
Regular (soluble)	0.5–1	2–3	3–6
Intermediate acting			
NPH (isophane)	2–4	4–10	10–16
Lente (insulin zinc suspension)	3–4	4–12	12–18
Long acting			
Ultralente (extended insulin zinc suspension)	6–10	10–16	18–20
Insulin glargine (analog)	2–4	Peakless	20–24
Combinations			
50% NPH, 50% regular	0.5–1	Dual	10–16
70% NPH, 30% regular	0.5–1	Dual	10–16
70% NPA, 30% aspart	<0.25	Dual	10–16
75% NPL, 25% lispro	≤0.25	Dual	10–16

*Per manufacturers' data; other data indicate equivalent pharmacodynamic effect (Plank J, Wutte A, Brunner G, Siebenhofer A, Semlitsch B, Sommer R, Hirschberger S, Pieber TR: Direct comparison of insulin aspart and insulin lispro in patients with type 1 diabetes. *Diabetes Care* 25:2053–2057, 2002).

understood may cause rates of absorption to vary by 20–40% from day to day in any one patient. In light of the many other variables influencing insulin pharmacokinetics, the clinician is cautioned against relying too heavily on textbook descriptions of insulin action. Health professionals should base therapy adjustments on actual glycemic values obtained from the patient's self-monitoring of blood glucose (SMBG).

Rapid- and short-acting insulins are relatively predictable on a day-to-day basis in onset and duration of action. Therefore, they can be adjusted on a 2- to 3-day observation period to normalize postprandial glucose values. Any change in the dose of intermediate-acting (NPH or lente) or long-acting (glargine or ultralente) insulin requires a 2- to 5-day observation period before further dose adjustment because of the relatively slow absorption and long duration of action of these insulins and because of day-to-day variability in food, activity, and stress.

The use of SMBG to map out a profile of blood glucose values is invaluable in assisting the physician, patient, and diabetes management team with therapy. Blood glucose levels should be measured before and after meals and during the night, particularly when initiating or intensifying insulin therapy or when seeking the cause of hypoglycemia or hyperglycemia. Routine frequency of monitoring should be based on mutually defined goals described in PHILOSOPHY AND GOALS.

Insulin Pens and Devices

Most of the current human insulins and insulin analogs are available in insulin cartridges and/or disposable pens (Table 3.1). Such devices aid the patient in insulin measurement and simplify insulin administration with minimal added cost to therapy. Several manufacturers of insulin pens and pen needles exist; some devices perform glucose monitoring in addition. Use of these devices will not only facilitate the adaptation to basal-bolus therapy but also enhance the compliance to intensive insulin therapy.

Mixing Insulins

Mixing insulin is still common, though declining, in the United States because of the slow adaptation to insulin pens. The action-prolonging substances in modified insulins (especially lente and ultralente) can sometimes affect the onset, peak, and duration of effectiveness of short- or rapid-acting insulin in a mixture. Generally, the longer the contact time between the two types of insulin and the larger the proportion of intermediate- or long-acting insulin in the mixture, the less rapid the absorption of the short- or rapid-acting insulin. Therefore, blood glucose levels fall at a slower rate, but the effect lasts longer.

It is not advisable to premix lente or ultralente with short- or rapid-acting insulin in the same syringe. Mixing any insulin with glargine is also not advised because of the formation of precipitants that occur on mixing. Mixing short- or rapid-acting insulin with NPH in the same syringe is an accepted and convenient way to produce differently timed pharmacologic actions with a single injection. Stable premixtures of intermediate- and short- or rapid-acting insulins in fixed proportion (e.g., 70% NPH/30% regular, 75% NPL/25% insulin lispro) are also available commercially. Premixed insulins are not suitable when daily variation in the dose of short-acting insulin is required, which is the case for most patients with type 1 diabetes.

TREATING NEWLY DIAGNOSED PATIENTS

Diagnosis and Stabilization

At diagnosis, initial objectives of therapy are eliminating symptomatic hyperglycemia (and concomitant fluid and electrolyte imbalance) while avoiding hypoglycemia. Therefore, glycemic targets should be approached gradually. Treatment should begin with ~0.6–0.75 unit/kg/day. However, during the first week of therapy, this amount can be expected to increase to an average of 1 unit/kg/day, because most patients are relatively insulin resistant at this time. This is particularly true for adolescents.

Immediately after diagnosis or after ketoacidosis has been resolved, therapy should begin with the insulin program that is planned to be used, e.g., twice-daily insulin injections or a "flexible" intensive insulin program consisting of preprandial or bolus insulin at each meal and basal insulin once or twice per day. It is preferable to start with the flexible basal-bolus insulin program at the outset instead of learning twice-daily insulin injections, a therapy that eventually fails. Although twice- or once-daily insulin may suffice for a short time in patients who retain some of their β-cell function, psychological acceptance of flexible intensive injection programs is easier for both patient and family if introduced as soon as possible after diagnosis, even if glycemic control could be adequate on a different program with fewer injections. Moreover, there is evidence from the Diabetes Control and Complications Trial (DCCT) that intensive exogenous insulin helps preserve β-cell function and should be given in adequate doses so that the patient does not need to utilize endogenous insulin for routine glycemic control.

Although not recommended, many clinicians start with a twice-daily program, to acquaint the patient with basic diabetes management principles, before initiating a flexible intensive program. When such is the case, about two-thirds of the insulin dose is given in the morning before breakfast, and one-third is given before supper. The two doses may consist of premixed insulins (sometimes the case for infants and very young children) or two doses of a mixture of rapid- or short- and intermediate-acting insulins. The prebreakfast dose consists of about two-thirds NPH (or lente) and one-third regular or insulin aspart or lispro. The presupper dose is usually divided into equal amounts of NPH (or lente) and regular insulin or insulin aspart or lispro.

Patients and families should be taught the technique of blood glucose monitoring at diagnosis. They should determine blood glucose levels repeatedly under professional supervision to ensure the reliability of the readings. Although premixed formulations (e.g., 70% NPH/30% regular; 75% NPL/25% insulin lispro) may work satisfactorily in some patients under very stable control, all patients should have supplies of short- or rapid-acting and longer-acting insulins for use when needed.

Honeymoon Phase

Within weeks after diagnosis there may be some recovery of β-cell function, and consequently, exogenous insulin requirements often decrease for weeks to months. This honeymoon phase of type 1 diabetes may be marked by the appearance of recurrent hypoglycemic reactions. A honeymoon phase occurs less frequently in younger children; it is more common in the late teenage years and in adults. During this period, insulin dosage must be appropriately reduced, occasionally to as little as 0.1–0.3 unit/kg/day. Not all patients exhibit a profound honeymoon phase, but some period of stability in blood glucose levels is common, with insulin requirements at 0.2–0.5 unit/kg/day. Evidence suggests that the honeymoon phase could be prolonged if blood glucose levels are kept in the near-normal range with basal/bolus therapy. There should not be an attempt to reduce insulin to the lowest dose possible nor to discontinue insulin. Instead, the patient should receive the highest dose that does not induce hypoglycemia.

Chronic Phase: Developing a Long-Term Treatment Plan

As the honeymoon period comes to an end with the progressive decrease of β-cell function, insulin requirements increase gradually over several months. Prepubertal children usually require between 0.6 and 0.9 unit/kg/day, and pubertal children may require up to 1.5 units/kg/day because of relative insulin resistance, increased caloric intake during rapid growth spurts, and changes in hormone secretory patterns. After puberty, insulin requirements should decrease to <1.0 unit/kg/day to prevent excessive weight gain. Dose requirements for pregnant patients vary with gestational duration and are discussed in Pregnancy (page 146).

Most physicians start patients with newly diagnosed type 1 diabetes on human insulin. Careful balance of caloric intake, activity, and insulin dose is required for an insulin regimen to be successful. It is most desirable to vary insulin doses to coincide with variations of food intake, activity, and prevailing blood glucose. On the other hand, if insulin dose is kept constant from day to day, food intake and activity should also be kept constant. The choice of insulin regimen should be based on individual characteristics, preferences, and habits, including age, stage of development, meal plans, and potential adherence to diabetes treatment. The diabetes management team should develop an acceptable and realistic treatment plan together with the patient. For example, an adolescent patient who is experiencing difficulties in following the treatment and has frequent episodes of hyperglycemia or ketoacidosis may have to be treated with two injections per day administered by a family member or visiting nurse until his or her problems are resolved. Switching to less frequent, longer-acting insulin injections ensures that at least the total insulin requirement is administered and may improve glucose control while avoiding ketoacidosis.

After the initial dose adjustments, ongoing long-term adjustments are made on the basis of daily repeated blood glucose measurements. Blood glucose levels should be monitored before meals and at bedtime every day and periodically between 3:00 and 4:00 a.m. (perhaps once per week). With time and practice, patients and families are able to make the adjustments with relative ease and become progressively independent of the diabetes management team. In addition to the long-term adjustments, insulin doses and waiting times between injections and food intake could be adjusted in response to high or low blood glucose levels, changes in food intake, activity level, or intercurrent illness. These adjustments can be made by patients who have been thoroughly trained and who can measure their blood glucose levels precisely.

Patient education is time-consuming but essential and should be conducted by a skilled diabetes management team working together with the patient and his or her family. Most patients require an initial period of instruction of 10–12 h, with periodic review and follow-up sessions every few months until both patient and family feel comfortable with their knowledge. Insulin regimens and blood glucose targets also should vary depending on the individual patient and should take into consideration the frequency and adherence to SMBG, the patient's ability to recognize and respond to hypoglycemic reactions, and the limitations imposed by what the patient and/or family are willing or ready to do. However, individualization should not prevent continued efforts toward the goal of achieving near-normoglycemia while avoiding severe hypoglycemia.

A frequent problem in the management of diabetes is the disappointment that sets in at the end of the honeymoon period when patients and parents of children with type 1 diabetes realize that the efforts invested in the treatment are not rewarded by the achievement of normoglycemia. Often, minor deviations from treatment or even no deviations at all result in unexplained fluctuations of blood glucose levels. Because these fluctuations are part of the nature of type 1 diabetes, even under the strictest and most flexible treatment conditions, such as with the use of multiple injections and insulin pumps, it is helpful at diagnosis to warn patients and families that the treatment of diabetes is imperfect and that blood glucose fluctuations are to be expected. Adequate explanations about the unpredictability of blood glucose levels and their relationship to daily variations of insulin absorption, food composition and absorption, and changes in the level of physical activity often help to prevent the development of feelings of guilt and incompetence that can plague patients and families. A useful attitude on the part of the diabetes management team is to stress the importance of overall blood glucose control rather than individual values, allowing for relatively wide fluctuations (70–160 mg/dl [3.9–8.9 mmol/l] preprandial and up to 200 mg/dl [11.1 mmol/l] postprandial), even when narrower glycemic targets are selected.

INSULIN REGIMENS

General Principles

Normal insulin secretion is characterized by continuous basal release, with superimposed bursts of additional insulin integrated precisely to the rise in blood glucose after food intake. Additionally, insulin is secreted into the portal vein and thus goes to the liver before entering the general circulation. Ideally, exogenous insulin treatment regimens should mimic all aspects of this pattern. Unfortunately, with the available means of treatment, this is not clinically possible. Therefore, insulin treatment regimens represent varying degrees of compromise to achieve near-normalization of blood glucose levels, one of the most important goals of diabetes management. Ideally, insulin regimens should have both basal and bolus components of normal insulin secretion.

Prandial or bolus insulin is best mimicked by administering rapid-acting (insulin lispro or aspart) or short-acting (regular) insulin before meals at the appropriate time, depending on the blood glucose level. Prandial insulin comprises ~50–60% of the total daily dose. Advantages of rapid-acting insulin analogs over human regular insulin are convenience (injection at or after a meal instead of 30 min premeal), better postprandial control, and reduced risk of postprandial hypoglycemia occurring 3–6 h postinjection. Disadvantages of rapid-acting analogs are cost and inability to cover snacks without another bolus injection of insulin.

Basal insulin secretion comprises ~40–50% of the total daily dose. It can be mimicked best by delivering short- or rapid-acting insulin continuously by an insulin pump (continuous subcutaneous insulin infusion [CSII]) or by giving long-acting insulin glargine once or twice a day. The basal insulin in CSII has the advantage of being variable and adjustable to cover the dawn rise in glucose levels (the dawn phenomenon) and decreased or discontinued in the case of exercise or hypoglycemia. Compared to NPH, lente, and ultralente, insulin glargine has the advantage of being relatively peakless, with onset being 1.5 h postinjection and mean duration of action being 23.5 h after several days of injections. As a result, clinical studies in type 1 diabetes have shown better fasting blood glucose with less nocturnal hypoglycemia than NPH once, twice, or four times daily. In ~20% of individuals, glargine lasts <20 h and may have to be given twice daily, usually in a 50:50 format. Disadvantages of glargine over NPH are that it is only a basal insulin and does not cover snacks without a bolus injection, is not mixable with other insulins in the same syringe, and is Category C in pregnancy and thus not recommended in pregnancy.

Traditionally, NPH, lente, and ultralente have been and still are used as basal insulins. If used, they should be given twice daily at breakfast and bedtime. The intermediate-acting insulins have an onset of action ~2 h after the injection and produce peak levels ~6–10 h after injection. Daytime NPH or lente provides basal hyperinsulinemia, and snacks may be needed to prevent hypoglycemia. Bedtime NPH or lente provides overnight basal hyperinsulinemia with peak serum insulins around breakfast time and thus reduces the risk of nocturnal hypoglycemia. Long-acting insulin is given once daily before breakfast or at bedtime or twice daily at breakfast and bedtime or at breakfast and supper. Disadvantages of ultralente are the marked intraindividual variation in absorption with resultant variable and often unpredictable glucose control.

Starting Insulin Requirement

The starting insulin dose is usually based on body weight. On average, a patient will eventually require anywhere between 0.4 to 1.0 unit/kg/day with higher amounts during puberty. It is best to start conservative at 0.5 unit/kg/day and increase insulin doses accordingly to SMBG readings.

Once-Daily Insulin

It is nearly impossible to adequately treat type 1 diabetes with once-daily insulin. However, among some adolescents and a few adults, a once-daily regimen, which almost always results in only an unacceptable level of glycemic control, may be the only outcome achievable without alienating the patient. Once-daily regimens are sometimes effective for short periods during the honeymoon phase, when residual insulin secretion is substantial, but are not recommended.

Although not recommended, this regimen uses a single morning injection of intermediate- or long-acting insulin, alone or in combination with short-acting (regular) insulin. The short-acting insulin has major action between breakfast and early afternoon, and its effect is reflected in the noon and presupper blood glucose levels. The NPH insulin has major action between midafternoon and bedtime, with some effect at night, and its effect is reflected in the bedtime and fasting glucose values. If forced to use this undesirable approach, one may start with three-quarters of the total dose as NPH and one-quarter as regular in young patients, and two-thirds NPH with one-third regular in adults. An extra dose of short- or rapid-acting insulin may be given before supper if blood glucose values are above the target. Patients on once-daily injection regimens commonly experience afternoon or evening hypoglycemia, often in combination with nocturnal hyperglycemia. Almost always, a major improvement in glycemic control will result from a change to even one of the two-injection regimens described below.

Whether a once-daily injection regimen is adopted at the request of the patient or because the physician believes that the patient will not accept more than one injection a day, it is almost always inadequate. Clinical and biochemical goals should always be reviewed with these patients, and sometimes a better understanding of the reasons for changing to more than a single morning injection leads to acceptance (see Philosophy and Goals, page 23).

Two or Three Injections Daily

The twice-daily "split-mixed" insulin regimen (Fig. 3.1) was the most commonly used treatment regimen before results of the DCCT. Morning short- or rapid-acting insulin (regular or insulin aspart/lispro) has major action between breakfast and lunch, and its effect is reflected in the prelunch blood glucose levels. Morning intermediate-acting (NPH or lente) insulin has major action between breakfast and supper, and its effect is reflected in the presupper blood glucose levels. Evening short-acting insulin has major action between supper and bedtime, and its effect is reflected in the bedtime tests. The evening intermediate-acting insulin has its major action overnight, and its effect is reflected in the blood glucose level on arising the next morning. The initial dose can be divided (based on % of total daily insulin) into a morning injection containing ~40% NPH and ~15% insulin aspart/lispro or regular at breakfast, plus an evening injection containing ~30% NPH and ~15% insulin aspart/lispro or regular at supper. In younger children, the proportions are closer to 80%/20% for both components.

The theoretical advantages of this regimen are *1)* the reduction of preprandial and postprandial hyperglycemia and *2)* the reduction of overnight and fasting glycemia. The most frequent and serious disadvantage of this regimen is that, in many patients, attempts to achieve fasting normoglycemia result in nocturnal hypoglycemia (from midnight to 8:00 a.m.) and early morning hyperglycemia (from 4:00 to 8:00 a.m., the dawn phenomenon). In these cases, it is better to move the intermediate-acting insulin to bedtime and thus reduce the peak effect of insulin from 2:00 to 4:00 a.m. and increase it at dawn (Fig. 3.1B). However, postprandial hyperglycemia is often not controlled without the risk of daytime hypoglycemia, and thus, an insulin injection at lunch or with an afternoon snack is often needed. Generally, it is not possible to achieve near-normal glycemic levels with two or three injections per day.

Multiple-Component Flexible Regimens

Basal insulin requirements account for ~50% of the patient's total daily dose. Basal insulin may be provided as glargine, NPH, lente, or ultralente insulin with multiple-dose insulin programs or as a basal infusion of regular or insulin aspart/lispro with CSII. The remaining ~50% is given as prandial insulin, using either rapid-acting insulin aspart/lispro or short-acting regular insulin, delivered before meals and/or snacks either by syringe, pen, or an insulin pump bolus. A typical starting distribution would be ~25% of the total daily dose as a short-acting insulin pulse before breakfast, ~10% before lunch, and ~20% before

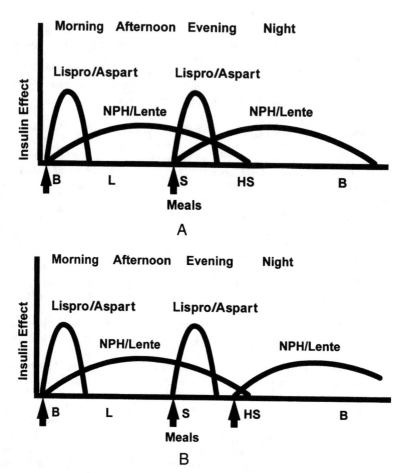

Figure 3.1 Schematic representation of idealized insulin effect provided by (A) "split-mixed" insulin regimen consisting of two daily injections of rapid-acting and intermediate-acting insulin given before breakfast and supper and (B) three daily injections with rapid-acting and intermediate-acting insulin before breakfast, rapid-acting insulin at supper, and intermediate-acting insulin at bedtime. B, breakfast; L, lunch; S, supper; HS, bedtime; *Arrow*, time of insulin injection, before meals.

supper. These prandial boluses are varied based on the carbohydrate content of the meal as well as the actual blood glucose determined by SMBG at that time.

A multiple-injection regimen features injections of regular insulin or insulin aspart/lispro preceding meals, coupled with longer-acting preparations that mimic basal insulin secretion. The most common regimen consists of premeal injections

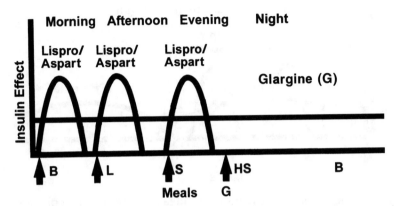

Figure 3.2 Schematic representation of idealized insulin effect provided by three daily injections with rapid-acting insulin at meals and once-daily insulin glargine at bedtime. B, breakfast; L, lunch; S, supper; HS, bedtime; *Arrow,* time of insulin injection.

(regular insulin or insulin aspart/lispro) plus glargine given at bedtime (Fig. 3.2). Glargine can also be given at supper or breakfast, and if needed, twice a day. Glargine cannot be mixed in the same syringe with other insulin preparations. Another alternative is the combination of premeal injections (regular insulin or insulin aspart/lispro) at breakfast, lunch, and supper, with NPH or lente at bedtime and with a small amount of NPH or lente before breakfast (Fig. 3.3) or at every meal.

The combination of premeal short- or rapid-acting insulin with bedtime glargine has been quite popular because *1)* it offers flexibility in meal size and timing, *2)* it is very easily understood by most patients because each period of the day has a well-defined insulin component, and *3)* the introduction of insulin pens has made it very convenient. Bedtime administration of glargine allows the easy titration of the fasting glucose to normal with minimal risk of nocturnal hypoglycemia. If bedtime or presupper glucoses are high with normal postlunch values and no afternoon snack, then consider the use of glargine twice a day. Another basal option is glargine only in the morning with titration to obtain the following fasting morning glucoses to be in the normal range. If this is not successful due either to daytime hypoglycemia or fasting hyperglycemia, then glargine must be given twice a day.

Continuous Subcutaneous Insulin Infusion (CSII)

The most precise way to mimic normal insulin secretion clinically is to use an insulin pump in a program of CSII (Fig. 3.4). Pump devices provide continuous insulin administration to normalize blood glucose levels throughout the 24-h period. Because insulin delivery is continuous, it can more or less mimic normal insulin secretion. The pump delivers microliter amounts of rapid- or short-

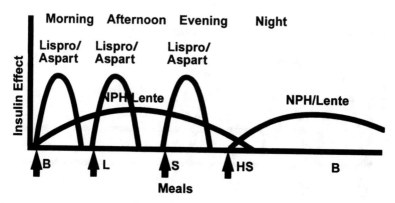

Figure 3.3 Schematic representation of idealized insulin effect provided by three daily injections with rapid-acting insulin at meals and two daily injections of intermediate-acting insulin at breakfast and at bedtime. B, breakfast; L, lunch; S, supper; HS, bedtime; *Arrow,* time of insulin injection.

acting insulin (insulin aspart/lispro or buffered regular) on a continual basis, thus replicating basal insulin secretion. The basal rate may be programmed to vary at times of diurnal variation in insulin sensitivity, if such variation results in disruption of glycemic control. Thus, the basal infusion rate may be programmed either to be decreased overnight to avert nocturnal hypoglycemia or to be increased to counteract the dawn phenomenon, which often results in hyperglycemia on awakening. Unique patterns of basal infusions may be needed by some patients, but most patients' circadian insulin requirements are met with one to three basal rates per day.

The pump may be activated before meals to provide increments of insulin as meal "boluses" whenever that meal or snack is consumed. This allows total flexibility in meal timing. If regular insulin is used, the meal boluses are given ~20–30 min before a meal. If insulin aspart/lispro is used, the meal boluses are given immediately before eating a meal. If a meal is skipped, the insulin bolus is omitted. If a meal is larger or smaller than usual, a larger or smaller insulin bolus is selected based on the carbohydrate content of the meal. Some pumps also offer variable bolus options including immediate delivery, square-wave delivery over a set amount of time (~2 h), or dual-wave delivery with both immediate and square-wave delivery together. Dual-wave delivery is useful for high-fat meals such as pizza and Mexican food, as well as for patients suspected of having gastroparesis. Frequent SMBG or the use of a continuous glucose monitoring system (CGMS) will help to determine the proper setting of the immediate and square-wave bolus. If the patient is anorexic or nauseous, the bolus can be delayed until following the meal (e.g., in early pregnancy or during illness). Thus, CSII patients have the potential of easily varying meal size and meal timing, as well as omitting meals, without sabotaging glycemic control.

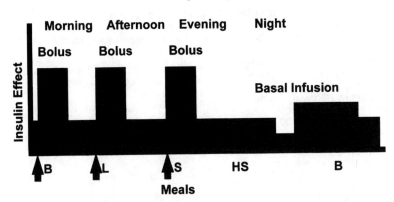

Figure 3.4 Schematic representation of idealized insulin effect provided by continuous subcutaneous insulin infusion (insulin pump) with insulin aspart/lispro. B, breakfast; L, lunch; S, supper; HS, bedtime. *Arrow,* time of insulin bolus, at meals.

The ability to program insulin pumps allows "suspension" of insulin delivery with increased physical activity, which serves to reduce the risk of exercise-related hypoglycemia. Caution should be exercised in suspending delivery of insulin aspart/lispro, because hyperglycemia may rapidly supervene if insulin delivery is interrupted for >2 h. Switching to a reduced temporary basal may be preferable. With regular insulin, delivery usually may be interrupted for 3 h without significant hyperglycemia emerging.

Infusion pumps are relatively small, lightweight, portable, battery-driven devices. The devices on the market have such features as alarms for low battery, blocked delivery, and empty reservoir. Other options found in some pumps include variable basal rates, preprogrammed boluses, and different bolus options. Newer advanced pumps have recently added correction bolus algorithms, carbohydrate counting algorithms, alerts to recommend SMBG tests and changing the infusion sets at specified times, and wireless connections to blood glucose meters. Most offer a quick-release device to remove the pump for such activities as swimming, contact sports, showering, sexual activity, or dressing.

Treatment with insulin pumps is extremely effective in improving glucose control in patients with type 1 diabetes, particularly those motivated patients most interested in meticulous glycemic control. Indications for CSII are listed in Table 3.3.

On initiating CSII therapy, the patient must receive instruction from the diabetes management team, including

- accurate monitoring of capillary blood glucose before each meal, at bedtime, and at mid-sleep

Table 3.3 Indications for Insulin Pump Therapy (CSII)

- Inadequate glycemic control, defined as:
  - A1C above target (>7.0% nonpregnant, >6.5% if planning pregnancy, >5.5% if pregnant)
  - Dawn phenomenon with fasting SMBG >140 mg/dl (8 mmol/l)
  - Marked variability in SMBG on a day-to-day basis
- History of severe hypoglycemia or hypoglycemia unawareness
- Need for flexibility in lifestyle (e.g., shift worker, traveler, or worker in safety-sensitive job)

- knowing safe blood glucose targets during the night and early morning (>80 mg/dl [>4.4 mmol/l]) to avoid hypoglycemia, the most frequent complication of intensive therapy
- learning strategies to reduce the risk of nocturnal hypoglycemia, if it ensues, including increasing the target fasting blood glucose to 100–140 mg/dl (5.6–7.8 mmol/l), decreasing the basal rate if 3:00 a.m. blood glucose levels are <80 mg/dl (<4.4 mmol/l), and daily measurements of blood glucose levels at bedtime followed by 15 g of carbohydrate if the values are ≤100 mg/dl (≤5.5 mmol/l)
- caring for infusion site with changes of the catheter every 2–3 days to avoid infection and inflammation
- understanding the urgency of changing the infusion set immediately in the event of hyperglycemia and troubleshooting the possibility of crimped cannula, leaking, or obstruction after correcting the problem
- knowing how to contact experienced medical personnel by phone 24 h per day, 7 days per week
- having the constant presence of a relative or friend until the patient becomes familiar with the pump

The initial programming of the pump is based on the total daily insulin dose of the previous regimen. Approximately 50% of the total dose is given as the basal rate, and the rest is divided between breakfast, lunch, supper, and snacks.

The patient is generally started with a single basal rate over a 24-h period. Bedtime snacks are not given until the basal rate is correct overnight. The basal rate is adjusted every second or third day on the basis of the blood glucose levels at bedtime, mid-sleep, and on rising until the desired blood glucose target is obtained. Increments should be in the order of 10–15% or 0.1 unit/h. In the case of nocturnal hypoglycemia, basal rate should be lowered starting 2–3 h before the time of the hypoglycemic event. Patients exhibiting the dawn phenomenon may require increased basal rates in the early morning hours starting 2–3 h before waking and lasting 4–6 h. Children may have a reverse dawn phenomenon requiring higher basal rates between 10:00 p.m. and 2:00 a.m. Basal rates are adjusted during the day only when meals are delayed or skipped and blood glucose levels rise or fall >30 mg/dl (>1.7 mmol/l) during that time.

Even when a patient's initial commitment persists, the use of pumps may be associated with various problems. These include local inflammation at catheter sites from infection or tape irritation, pump breakdown and/or malfunction, forgetting to refill reservoirs on time, or forgetting to give meal boluses. Luer lock leaks or a crimped soft cannula may interfere with insulin delivery, with resultant hyperglycemia, ketonemia, and diabetic ketoacidosis.

Appropriate education in troubleshooting hyperglycemia, hypoglycemia, as well as other problems must be provided. The introduction of more flexible infusion sets (which reduce local irritation) and the development of better pump insulins (human buffered regular, and aspart) to minimize insulin precipitation and resulting catheter obstruction have helped. More recently, the development of programmable software to calculate the correction bolus, determine the bolus for a set amount of carbohydrates, and alerts for SMBG tests and reservoir changes will obviously minimize many of the prior problems associated with pump therapy. The major disadvantage remains the inexorable need for SMBG values, four to six times per day. This will be eliminated only if reliable continuous glucose sensors can be developed. These continuous sensors in turn will then be linked with mechanical insulin delivery devices.

OPTIMIZING BLOOD GLUCOSE CONTROL

Physiologic insulin secretion in nondiabetic individuals involves *1*) meal-related increased insulin secretion initiated by neural and gut factors before the hyperglycemic stimulus that is responsible for tissue uptake and storage of nutrients, followed by a rapid return of insulin secretion to the baseline level, and *2*) basal insulin secretion between meals and during the night to regulate amino acids and fatty acids in the fasting state and to prevent excessive fasting gluconeogenesis. It is presumed that only an artificial β-cell with continuous glucose monitoring and the administration of short-acting insulin into the portal circulation can replicate the function of the normal pancreas.

Proper diabetes management has the goal of approaching normal blood glucose levels without severe hypoglycemia. The preprandial plasma blood glucose levels will most likely be outside the desired premeal values of 90–130 mg/dl (5.0–7.2 mmol/l) and peak postprandial values of <180 mg/dl (<10.0 mmol/l). Safe middle-of-the-night values are in the range of 70–120 mg/dl (3.9–6.7 mmol/l). These targets are difficult to maintain safely except under very intensive programs with selected patients.

In the DCCT, the goals of intensive treatment were to reduce glycated hemoglobin (A1C) to <6% and to maintain this difference for up to 10 yr. In the trial, 44% of patients achieved that goal at least once during the study. However, <5% of patients maintained an average value in that range. In response to the DCCT results, the American Diabetes Association recommended that "patients should aim for the best level of glucose control they can achieve without placing themselves at undue risk for hypoglycemia or other hazards associated with tight control." Therapy must be individualized. If the resources are available and the patient is willing, reasonable outcomes include mean plasma glucose of 140–160 mg/dl (7.8–8.9 mmol/l) and A1C values of 6.5–7.5%.

The implications of the DCCT findings are that optimal treatment should be offered to all patients. That means a progression from twice-daily to multiple injections or the insulin pump depending on the response to treatment and the patient's ability and willingness to comply.

To achieve near-normal glycemic levels, it is advisable to use algorithms for adjusting both the insulin dose and the timing of the meal. Insulin algorithms are protocols for adjusting the dose and timing of insulin and meals based on regularly monitored blood glucose levels. They also allow patients to adjust insulin dose in relation to amount and composition of food and exercise. Although flexible, such regimens tend to place a great demand on both patient and physician. Tables 3.4 and 3.5 present an example of a step-by-step approach to improving and intensifying therapy. The efficacy of insulin algorithms is predicated on

- reasonable and consistent adherence to carbohydrate counting
- adjustment of insulin based on SMBG

Table 3.4 Evaluating Suboptimally Controlled Diabetes

- Increase frequency of SMBG. Patient should measure blood glucose 5 times/day (fasting, premeal, at bedtime, and during the night). Blood glucose values 70–140 mg/dl (3.9–7.8 mmol/l) are considered good; repeated values outside this range are unacceptable and require action.
- Identify the probable cause of high or low blood glucose values. Consider the following:
  - Exercise or activity that is irregular or erratic
  - Snacks for which insulin is not given
  - Inconsistency in meal timing and/or size
  - Emotional or psychiatric problems, including stress
  - Alcohol or drug problems
  - Occult chronic infection or other inflammatory condition
  - Problems with insulin administration—inaccuracy, site selection, timing
  - Problems with SMBG—damaged strips, a noncalibrated meter, dishonest or incomplete recording
  - Insulin reactions—treatment of undocumented hypoglycemia, overtreatment, hypoglycemia unawareness
  - Deliberate noncompliance with regimen—insulin omission to lose weight and eating disorders
- Note recurring glycemic patterns. Factors such as the following may be operative:
  - Fasting hyperglycemia: dawn phenomenon, rebound hyperglycemia, waning insulin effect
  - Late-afternoon hypoglycemia: morning intermediate-acting insulin dose too large
  - Overnight hypoglycemia: evening intermediate- or long-acting insulin dose too large or injected too early
  - Erratic glycemic patterns may result from overinsulinization, antibody binding of insulin, or gastrointestinal motility disorders
- Alter therapy appropriately (Table 3.5).

Table 3.5 Steps for Optimizing Therapy

- Obtain baseline (2–7 days) blood glucose profiles, A1C, and fasting lipids as well as baseline ophthalmologic and renal parameters. If the A1C value does not correspond to the blood glucose values, be certain that the patient does not have a hemoglobinopathy or hemolytic problem that precludes accurate assessment of mean blood glucose long term.
- If patient is on a 1- or 2-injection regimen and profiles indicate hyperglycemia or nighttime hypoglycemia, start multiple daily insulin regimen.
- Adjust meals and snacks to optimize timing, calories, and source of carbohydrate.
- Instruct patient to perform SMBG 4–5 times daily (prebreakfast, prelunch, presupper, bedtime, and nighttime) and to keep daily logbook of insulin doses and SMBG results. Calibrate meter and verify accuracy of technique by direct observation, provide patient with meter that has accessible memory.
- Instruct patient to identify and record probable cause of high or low glucose values (e.g., overeating, late meal, skipped snack, excess activity, illness).
- Schedule office visits more frequently (e.g., every 1–4 wk) for detailed discussion and review of SMBG results, feedback from staff, and help with problem solving.
- Increase SMBG to include postprandial periods and several measurements during the night, particularly if A1C is discrepantly higher than premeal glucoses would indicate. Examine SMBG pattern for subtle asymptomatic hypoglycemia or nocturnal hypoglycemia (with or without subsequent posttreatment hyperglycemia) as well as waning insulin effect.
- Adjust short- or rapid-acting insulin doses according to individually constructed algorithms. Adjust insulin-to-carbohydrate ratio according to blood glucose values. All doses must be individualized for each patient. Use postprandial SMBG to recheck algorithm efficacy for correcting high or low glucose values toward 100 mg/dl (5.6 mmol/l).
- If goals remain unmet, verify that dietary and SMBG adherence and contact with staff are optimal. If these are problems, mutually redefine objectives to improve adherence in a nonjudgmental manner.
- Use of a continuous glucose monitoring system or similar system (GlucoWatch) should be considered if glycemic targets and goals are not met.
- Consider insulin pump therapy if glycemic goals are not met, major hypoglycemia or hypoglycemia unawareness exists, or flexibility in lifestyle is needed.

  - injecting insulin at the meal
  - a regular pattern of activity and willingness to make adjustments for unscheduled activities

Algorithms are used to correct for a given glucose value or to adjust insulin dosing for in anticipation of any blood glucose–altering factors, e.g., increased carbohydrate intake, most intercurrent stress, or changing physical activity.

Timing of Meals

If using regular insulin, it is preferable to give the insulin injection 20–30 min before meals so that plasma insulin levels are optimal for glucose disposal. If using insulin aspart/lispro, the injections are given just before eating. In very young children or persons with nausea, for whom it is not possible to estimate meal intake before eating, insulin aspart/lispro may be given after the meal.

Insulin-to-Carbohydrate Ratios

Patients with type 1 diabetes should be encouraged to learn carbohydrate counting and to calculate their insulin-to-carbohydrate ratio (I:C) to enhance flexibility in their diet and improve postprandial glucose control. The I:C can vary between 1 unit insulin/5 g carbohydrate to 1 unit insulin/25 g carbohydrate. To determine this ratio, the patient can either *1*) eat a fixed amount of carbohydrates with a meal, adjust the premeal insulin to obtain adequate postmeal glucose control, then determine the ratio, or *2*) start with an estimated ratio and adjust it accordingly to obtain adequate postmeal control. The I:C can be determined by a statistically established formula initially: I:C is equal to 2.8 times body weight in pounds (BW#) divided by the total daily dose of insulin (TDD). Therefore, I:C = 2.8 × BW#/TDD. Subsequently, the I:C can be adjusted by ≥1 g carbohydrate at a time based on analysis of postprandial glucose records. The I:C is usually the same at all meals but may be lower in the morning because of insulin resistance at that time. I:C can also change when there are changes in body weight or the total daily insulin dose.

Correction Bolus Algorithms (Compensatory Supplements of Insulin)

All patients on insulin should be provided with correction bolus algorithms to correct out-of-range glucose values. To do this, the insulin sensitivity, or correction factor (CF), must be determined for each patient. The insulin CF is defined as the number of mg/dl (mmol/l) the blood glucose will drop over a 2- to 4-h period following administration of 1 unit rapid- or short-acting insulin. Once this factor is determined, a corrective bolus or supplemental dose can be estimated and added to the normal premeal dose or can be given at other times to correct hyperglycemia.

The CF can be determined by using the "1700 rule," in which CF = 1700/TDD. For example, if a patient's TDD is 50 units insulin, the CF = 1700/50 = 35. In this case, 1 unit insulin should lower the patient's blood glucose level by 35 mg/dl (2 mmol/l). The CF can be used to calculate an individual's supplemental or correction bolus dose, where

correction dose = (actual blood glucose [BG] – midtarget BG)/CF

For most people, midtarget blood glucose is 100 mg/dl (5.5 mmol/l). However, patients prone to hypoglycemia may have a higher target (120 mg/dl [6.7 mmol/l]), and pregnant patients may have a lower target (80 mg/dl [4.4 mmol/l]). The correction dose is added to the premeal dose to optimize postmeal glucose levels. A patient's CF and correction dose are adjusted upon review of the SMBG records. The correction dose is also used in sick-day management for correcting hyperglycemia. Because of overlapping dosing effect when insulin is given again in less than 4 h, the target glucose should be increased to 140 when dosing at 2 h, i.e.,

correction dose = (BG – 140)/CF

Glycemic Targets and Insulin Adjustments

Adjustments of the insulin doses are made on the basis of SMBG measurements and are aimed at achieving target blood glucose values. Target glucose values are individualized based on the patient's ability to detect hypoglycemia and his or her current state of health. In most cases, targets are the normal values of a person without diabetes. If a child or a person has a proven problem coping with hypoglycemia, the target may be set higher. If pregnant, the target is set toward normal values for a pregnant woman without diabetes. Suggested glycemic targets are listed in Table 3.6.

Adjustments of insulin should be made with care to avoid hypoglycemia and overinsulinization. Dose adjustments should not surpass 1–2 units (decreases or increases) and should be made only when patterns of out-of-range glucose levels occur at the same time of day and are not attributed to transient changes in activity, food intake, or erroneous insulin injection. Ideally, adjustments upward should be made every 2–3 days for short- or rapid-acting insulin and every 3–5 days for long-acting insulin until the desired blood glucose targets are achieved. Adjustments downward should be made the next day for unexplained hypoglycemia, especially if severe.

There are different ways to achieve treatment targets. One method is to change the basal insulin to normalize the morning blood glucose level while avoiding hypoglycemia at 1:00–3:00 a.m. Basal insulin during the day can best be adjusted when the patient delays or skips a meal and no food intake has occurred for a minimum of 4 h. Bolus insulin is adjusted based on the postmeal or next premeal glucose values. Generally, the adequacy of prebreakfast rapid- or short-acting insulin is judged by the postbreakfast and/or prelunch blood glucose level, the adequacy of prelunch rapid- or short-acting insulin is judged by the postlunch and/or presupper blood glucose level, and the adequacy of presupper rapid- or short-acting insulin is judged by the postsupper and/or bedtime blood glucose level. Once blood glucose levels are normalized postmeal after a known amount of carbohydrates for that meal, an I:C can be calculated for that mealtime. The I:C is often the same for all times of day but can be lower in the morning due to higher insulin resistance at that time (See Nutrition).

Correction bolus algorithms are also adjusted if the glycemic response does not bring the glucose into the desired range. If the glycemic response consistently

Table 3.6 Suggested Glycemic Targets for Type 1 Diabetes in mg/dl (mmol/l)

Patient status	Premeal	Peak postprandial
Healthy	70–140 (4–8)	<160 (<9)
Prone to hypoglycemia or child or elderly	90–160 (5–9)	<180 (<10)
Pregnant	60–90 (3.5–5)	<120 (<6.5)

remains above target range, the insulin CF is lowered. If the glycemic response is too great and the glucose falls below target range, the insulin CF is increased.

All of the possible treatment options should be individualized according to meal plan, exercise, and lifestyle requirements. SMBG should be used frequently to profile glycemic values and to adjust therapy. Additionally, it is paramount that all treatment goals be mutually agreed on by the patient and the diabetes management team. Intensive therapy with multiple insulin injections or insulin pumps must be approached with knowledge and caution. All forms of intensive therapy require high degrees of commitment on the part of the patient, the family, and the diabetes management team. Dedication, knowledge, and time commitments are the rule. Demands of insulin pumps often require even more rigorous adherence to SMBG and other aspects of management and careful coordination by a team of experienced professionals. Because of the complexity of this problem, patients who are intent on achieving optimal glycemic control are best managed with an experienced team that includes a nurse trained in diabetes control, an endocrinologist or diabetes specialist, a dietitian, and a psychosocial counselor.

Barriers to Adherence

Even with initial commitment to intensified insulin therapy from the patient and diabetes management team, problems can arise. Many patients are eager to intensify therapy, but they must realize the commitment required. When the goals of the patient and the diabetes management team are not congruent, attempts at intensive insulin therapy are problematic.

A1C determinations inconsistent with SMBG meter memory download reports may have a physiologic explanation. In the past, such discrepancies, when documented only from patient records, were attributed to dishonesty and psychological problems, and often they may have been. Now, that problem can also be due to the memory chip in the meter.

COMMON PROBLEMS IN LONG-TERM THERAPY

Problems with insulin therapy arise regardless of the insulin regimen, and they must be addressed. Detecting and eliminating patterns of hypoglycemia and hyperglycemia are the cornerstone of caring for patients with diabetes. This is as true for the individual with diabetes of several years' duration as for the newly diagnosed patient.

Recurrent moderate or severe hypoglycemic reactions signal the need for evaluation of the insulin regimen, eating patterns, and other lifestyle factors (e.g., alcohol consumption). Exceptionally low A1C levels may identify patients at risk for moderate and/or severe hypoglycemia. Some patients have diminished symptoms of impending hypoglycemia (hypoglycemia unawareness) and, thus, suffer from recurrent hypoglycemic reactions and/or hypoglycemic seizures. In patients with hypoglycemia unawareness, blood glucose targets must be increased, and insulin pump therapy should be strongly considered.

Fasting hyperglycemia may occur in conjunction with high or low blood glucose values. If SMBG between 2:00 and 4:00 a.m. reveals nocturnal hypoglycemia, rebound hyperglycemia (Somogyi effect) may be operative, although blood glucose levels >200 mg/dl (>11.1 mmol/l) usually do not occur unless food is given to treat hypoglycemia. In this case, a decrease in evening intermediate- or long-acting insulin is needed. However, if no nocturnal hypoglycemia can be documented, inadequate insulin from 4:00 to 9:00 a.m. may be causative. This should be addressed with either an increase in presupper or bedtime insulin or a change from a presupper injection to a bedtime injection schedule. If this fails, insulin pump therapy needs to be considered with appropriate titration of overnight basal rates.

Inconsistencies in food intake and/or activity, often associated with psychosocial factors, can be causes of unacceptable day-to-day glucose control and elevated A1C levels. Other factors that may contribute to glycemic irregularities are listed in Table 3.4. Additional problems of insulin therapy, including changes in insulin absorption or sensitivity, surgery, hypoglycemia, and insulin allergy are discussed in subsequent parts of this chapter or in other chapters.

Once the sources of hypoglycemia and hyperglycemia have been eliminated, further efforts to tighten control may require continuous glucose sensing to determine the cause.

INSULIN ALLERGY

Allergic reactions to insulin are increasingly rare with the widespread use of human insulin. However, patients of all ages, particularly those with known atopic diseases, may exhibit local or systemic allergy to human insulin itself, protamine in NPH, the zinc used in the lente insulins, or the low pH of glargine insulin.

Some allergic-type reactions may be transient or artifactual. Burning, itching, and hives at injection sites may result from improper injection technique (intradermal rather than subcutaneous injection or injection of cold insulin) or from localized allergic phenomena.

If symptoms do not resolve and the patient's injection technique is sound, a change from one brand or type to another may be in order. True anaphylaxis or severe asthma, although rare, occurs occasionally and should be treated according to well-established protocols (e.g., antihistamines, epinephrine). If changing insulin type does not result in improvement, antihistamines can be prescribed. If atopic phenomena continue or if systemic symptoms occur, consultation with a diabetologist is recommended for alternative approaches, including insulin desensitization.

SPECIAL CONSIDERATIONS

Exercise

Because physical exercise offers numerous health benefits, it should be encouraged in every patient with diabetes. In anticipation of the glucose-lowering effects of exercise, e.g., 30–45 min of moderate to vigorous physical activity, it may be necessary to increase carbohydrate intake or decrease the insulin dose to avoid hypoglycemia during or after exercise. Exercise-related hypoglycemia results from increased glucose uptake and utilization by the exercising muscle. Exercise increases muscle insulin sensitivity before and after exercise and decreases stimulation of hepatic glucose release secondary to exogenous insulin. In the case of prolonged exercise (lasting >1–2 h), it is necessary to reduce the insulin dose because hypoglycemia can occur many hours after exercise. General guidelines for avoiding exercise-related hypoglycemia are given in Table 3.7.

- A decrease in prebreakfast rapid- or short-acting insulin is recommended if exercise is done within 3 h of breakfast.
- Decrease prelunch rapid- or short-acting insulin and/or morning NPH or lente insulin for exercise occurring in the late morning or early afternoon.
- Decrease presupper rapid- or short-acting insulin in anticipation of exercise occurring after supper.

Management During Acute Illnesses

The increased secretion of counterregulatory hormones and decreased activity even in the face of reduced caloric intake or vomiting may increase insulin requirements. Blood glucose and urine or blood ketone levels should be tested frequently (e.g., every 1–4 h or each time the patient urinates). The physician should be contacted immediately for advice if prior written guidelines are not known by the patient or family member. The following guidelines, based on whether the patient is able to take food or liquids by mouth, are useful for managing a patient during an illness.

An illness not accompanied by nausea or vomiting (e.g., minor infection or trauma requiring bed rest). If activity is normal, give the usual dose of basal

---

Table 3.7 General Guidelines for Avoiding Exercise-Induced Hypoglycemia in Insulin-Treated Patients

- Measure blood glucose before, during, and after exercise
- Unplanned exercise should be preceded by extra carbohydrate, e.g., 15–30 g per 30 min exercise; insulin may need to be decreased after exercise
- If exercise is planned, insulin dosages must be decreased before and after exercise according to the exercise intensity and duration as well as the personal experience of the individual with diabetes; insulin dose reductions may amount to 50–90% of daily insulin requirements
- During exercise, easily absorbable carbohydrate may need to be consumed
- After exercise, extra carbohydrate may be necessary and may be added to meals and snacks
- Athletes and those who exercise for fitness need specific instructions and training on self-management skills for exercise

Adapted from Berger M: Adjustment of insulin and oral agent therapy. In *Handbook of Exercise and Diabetes*. Ruderman N, Devlin JT, Schneider SH, Kriska A, Eds. Alexandria, VA, American Diabetes Association, 2002, p. 374.

insulin plus a correction bolus every 2–4 h as needed according to the blood glucose and ketone tests. If able to drink or eat, give, in addition to the correction bolus, the meal bolus insulin to cover the carbohydrate consumed. If an I:C is not known, give ~1–1.5 units insulin for every 15 g carbohydrate consumed.

If activity is reduced and the patient is confined to bed, caloric intake should be reduced by approximately one-third. The reduction in caloric intake compensates for the inactivity. The insulin adjustment is the same as for an illness without bed rest.

An illness accompanied by nausea, vomiting, or marked anorexia. Blood glucose and urine or blood ketones should be measured as soon as possible and every 2–4 h until the illness or situation has resolved. The insulin dose must never be omitted, because this could lead to ketoacidosis. If glucose is >240 mg/dl (13 mmol/l) and ketones are large, the patient should give a correction bolus by syringe and proceed to the emergency room to receive treatment for probable diabetic ketoacidosis. If glucose is >240 mg/dl (13 mmol/l) and ketones are not large, the patient can take a correction bolus every 2–4 h and drink noncaloric fluids until the situation has resolved. If on CSII, the infusion set and tubing must be changed. If the glucose is <240 mg/dl (13 mmol/l) and ketones are large, the patient can take a correction bolus every 2–4 h and consume caloric fluids as tolerated until the situation is resolved. When in doubt or the situation is not resolving, the patient should contact the health care provider.

In patients who have residual insulin or in very young children, it may be advantageous to omit the basal insulin (glargine, NPH, or lente) in the morning and switch to a more flexible multiple-injection regimen using injections of rapid- or short-acting insulin at breakfast, lunch, and supper, determined with an algorithm scale (in doses commensurate to the blood glucose tests and the presence or absence of ketonuria), plus basal insulin (glargine, NPH, or lente) at bedtime (~25% of the total daily insulin dose). If the patient is well by noon, one-half of the usual total daily dose of basal insulin is given together with short- or rapid-acting insulin. If the patient is not eating or drinking and fasting blood glucose level is normal, the dose of basal insulin may have to be reduced. Extra doses of short- or rapid-acting insulin given as correction boluses may be necessary every 4–6 h in the case of hyperglycemia. The meal plan should be replaced by "regular" (not "diet") soft drinks, fruit juice, or sweetened tea, 2–4 oz/h for children and 4–6 oz/h for adults.

Vomiting that occurs after administration of the usual morning dose of insulin. Sips of sugar-containing fluids should be given every 20–30 min to maintain blood glucose levels between 100 and 180 mg/dl (5.67 and 10.0 mmol/l). If vomiting persists and blood glucose level falls <100 mg/dl (<5.6 mmol/l), the patient may have to be taken to the hospital for intravenous glucose therapy. A subcutaneous injection of glucagon should be given at home before departing if the patient lives some distance from the hospital.

Whenever blood glucose level is >240 mg/dl (>13.3 mmol/l) and there is moderate or large ketonuria, the physician should be advised immediately or the patient should be brought to the emergency room, because this could reflect impending ketoacidosis. Repeated vomiting lasting more than 4–6 h or accompanied by high fever, abdominal pain, severe headache, or drowsiness may require that the patient be evaluated by a physician to ascertain whether he or she has a serious infection, appendicitis, meningitis, or other condition requiring antibiotics, surgery, or intensive medical care in a hospital setting.

Treatment of Diabetes in Infants

Transient neonatal diabetes can occur in newborn infants. These babies usually suffer from severe intrauterine malnutrition and, therefore, are small for their gestational age. They are hypoinsulinemic, fail to release insulin in response to any of the standard secretagogues, and must be treated with exogenous insulin with doses up to 1–2 units/kg/day. Insulin requirements are best established by starting a continuous intravenous insulin infusion at rates that provide at least 0.5 unit/kg/day. Insulin treatment is simplified by using diluted insulins (e.g., a solution containing 10 units/ml) so that inadvertent overdoses do not occur. It is very important to dilute the insulin with diluents received directly from the manufacturer. In most cases, β-cell function develops sometime between 6 and 12 weeks of age. It is thought that there is a delay in the development of normal β-cell growth and differentiation. These children commonly do well after the newborn period and do not appear to be at increased risk of developing type 1 diabetes at a later age. Islet cell antibodies are usually absent.

Type 1 diabetes can start in infancy or during the neonatal period. The treatment is similar to that described for the infant with neonatal hyperglycemia. Insulin requirements vary, and care of these patients should be supervised by an experienced specialist. Infants usually respond fairly well to twice-daily regimens with minimal or no short-acting insulin required. One of the problems found in these usually malnourished infants is that, because of the poor amount of subcutaneous fat, insulin injections are inadvertently given intramuscularly, and therefore, the duration of action is relatively unpredictable. If that is the case, an extra dose of intermediate-acting insulin should be added or insulin pump therapy should be considered.

Local Reactions

Lipohypertrophy at the injection site is the most common local complication of insulin therapy. It is thought to occur as a result of insulin stimulation of fat cell growth; the exact incidence is unknown. Lipoatrophy is rare with human insulin. If it does occur, changing brands of insulin may help. If either lipohypertrophy or lipoatrophy occur, rotation of injection sites with avoidance of the affected sites is recommended.

Insulin Resistance

Immunological insulin resistance due to antibodies to insulin is exceedingly rare, particularly since the introduction of purified insulins and human insulin. If it is suspected in a patient with unexplained severe insulin resistance, i.e., >2 units/kg/day after correction of ketosis with intravenous insulin, insulin antibody titers should be obtained in a reliable research laboratory. If positive, change in insulin brands and type of insulin should be considered. If problems persist, such patients should be seen by a consultant diabetologist experienced in the assessment and management of complex problems. Patients with insulin resistance due to high insulin antibodies sometimes improve with corticosteroid treatment or other immune suppression therapy. Apparent insulin resistance is much more likely to occur as the result of the patient's not taking insulin as prescribed or using insulin that has precipitated or aggregated from excessive shaking or heating.

CONCLUSION

Type 1 diabetes is characterized by a progressive decline of insulin secretion until its disappearance 1–5 yr after diagnosis. Thus, people with type 1 diabetes are dependent on insulin to survive. Insulin therapy is the most important aspect of the treatment of type 1 diabetes. However, insulin administration should always be coupled with SMBG. In this way, insulin therapy can be adjusted safely and effectively and individualized to age, lifestyle, eating habits, state of health, and physical activity. Effective insulin therapy helps the patient avoid extreme metabolic crises, such as hypo- and hyperglycemia, and achieve good glycemic control most of the time.

BIBLIOGRAPHY

Ahern JAH, Boland EA, Doane R, Ahern JJ, Rose P, Vincent M, Tamborlane WV: Insulin pump therapy in pediatrics: a therapeutic alternative to safely lower HbA1c levels across all age groups. *Pediatr Diabetes* 3:10–15, 2002

American Diabetes Association: *Intensive Diabetes Management.* 3rd ed. Klingensmith GJ, Ed. Alexandria, VA, American Diabetes Association, 2003

American Diabetes Association: *Practical Insulin: A Handbook for Prescribers.* Alexandria, VA, American Diabetes Association, 2002

Armstrong DU, King AB: Basal insulin: continuous glucose monitoring reveals less overnight hypoglycemia with continuous subcutaneous insulin infusion than with glargine (Abstract). *Diabetes* 51 (Suppl. 2):A92, 2002

Bode BW, Tamborlane WV, Davidson PC: Insulin pump therapy in the 21st century. *Postgrad Med* 111:69–77, 2002

Bolderman K: *Putting Your Patients on the Pump.* Alexandria, VA, American Diabetes Association, 2002

Bruttomesso D, Pianta A, Crazzola D, Scaldaferri E, Lora L, Guarneri G, Mongillo A, Gennaro R, Miola M, Moretti M, Confortin L, Beltramello GP, Pais M, Baritusso A, Casiglia E, Tienga A: Continuous subcutaneous insulin infusion (CSII) in the Veneto region: efficacy, acceptability, and quality of life. *Diabet Med* 19:628–634, 2002

Cersosimo E, Jornsay D, Arce C, Rieff M, Feldman E, DeFronzo R: Improved clinical outcomes with intensive insulin pump therapy in type 1 diabetes. (Abstract). *Diabetes* 51 (Suppl. 2):A128, 2002

Davidson PC, Hebblewhite HR, Bode BW, Richardson PL, Steed RD, Welch NS, Johnson J: Statistical estimates for CSII parameters: carbohydrate-to-insulin ratio (CIR); correction factor (CF); and basal insulin. *Diabetes Technol Ther* 5:A28, 2003

DeVries JH, Snoek FJ, Kostense PJ, Masurel N, Heine RJ: A randomized trial of continuous subcutaneous insulin infusion and intensive injection therapy in type 1 diabetes for patients with long-standing poor glycemic control. *Diabetes Care* 25:2074–2080, 2002

Lepore G, Dodesini AR, Nosari I, Trevisan R: Both continuous subcutaneous insulin infusion and a multiple daily insulin injection regimen with glargine as basal insulin are equally better than traditional multiple daily insulin injection treatment. *Diabetes Care* 26:1321–1322, 2003

Linkeschova R, Raoul M, Bott U, Berger M, Spraul M: Less severe hypoglycaemia, better metabolic control, and improved quality of life in type 1 diabetes mellitus with continuous subcutaneous insulin infusion (CSII) therapy: an observational study of 100 consecutive patients followed for a mean of 2 years. *Diabetic Med* 19:746–751, 2002

Litton J, Rice A, Friedman N, Oden J, Lee MM, Freemark M: Insulin pump therapy in toddlers and preschool children with type 1 diabetes mellitus. *J Pediatr* 141:490-495, 2002

Rudolph JW, Hirsch IB: Assessment of therapy with continuous subcutaneous insulin infusion in an academic diabetes clinic. *Endocrine Pract* 8:401–405, 2002

Santiago JV, White N: Diabetes in childhood and adolescence. In *International Textbook of Diabetes Mellitus*. 2nd ed. Alberti KGMM, Zimmet P, DeFronzo RA, Eds. Chichester, UK, Wiley, 1997, p. 1095–1122

Skyler JS: Insulin therapy in type 1 diabetes mellitus. In *Current Therapy of Diabetes Mellitus*. DeFronzo RA, Ed. St. Louis, MO, Mosby, 1998, p. 36–49

Wolpert H (Ed.): *Smart Pumping for People with Diabetes: A Practical Approach to Mastering the Insulin Pump*. Alexandria, VA, American Diabetes Association, 2002

MONITORING

Monitoring, performed by patients and by their diabetes management teams, is an integral feature of diabetes care. Specifically, results of blood glucose monitoring are useful in preventing hypoglycemia and adjusting insulin, diet, and exercise so that target blood glucose levels are achieved. Additionally, testing for urine or blood ketones provides an early warning sign of impending ketoacidosis.

PATIENT-PERFORMED MONITORING

Patients can manage their diabetes effectively and safely only if they are able to perform SMBG. In certain circumstances (infants, young children, hospitalized or incapacitated patients), monitoring may be performed by family members or health care providers.

In the past, the mainstay of diabetes monitoring was urine glucose testing. This method has distinct limitations and, therefore, is now considered obsolete. However, if after repeated explanations about its disadvantages the patient refuses to perform blood glucose testing, urine glucose testing is better than no testing at all to prevent excessive hyperglycemia.

SMBG is a direct method of testing plasma glucose that allows patients to determine their glucose levels anywhere (at home, school or work or while hospitalized) and to adjust therapy on the basis of accurate and timely results. To perform SMBG, a drop of blood is obtained from a fingertip or alternative site by use of a sharp lancet, usually with the aid of an automatic spring-loaded puncturing device. The blood is then applied to a chemically impregnated or electrochemical strip, and after a specified time, the result is quantitated and often stored in a meter.

Alternative site testing is available with some meters that need only a small amount of blood (<1 ml). Such testing, usually performed on the forearm but can also be done at other sites (hand, thigh), is reliable and correlates well with fingerstick testing in the premeal or fasting state but can have up to a 15- to 30-min lag if testing is done postmeal. Therefore, it is recommended that patients be aware of this lag and not make decisions solely based on alternative testing done postmeal. If in doubt regarding the value, verify the reading with fingerstick measurement.

Many commercially available strips and meters have been evaluated and are relatively reliable and reasonably accurate. Lists of SMBG products are found in the *Resource Guide*, published annually in the January issue of *Diabetes Forecast*, the American Diabetes Association's magazine. With appropriate education, most patients can perform the technique successfully. However, office return demonstrations of the patient's skills and the use of quality control techniques at home are essential. Patients should be encouraged to bring their meters to every office visit to assess their accuracy. Inaccurate measurements can be more dangerous than no measurements at all.

Frequency of SMBG

The frequency and timing of glucose monitoring should be dictated by the particular needs and goals of the patient. If the goal is to obtain near-normal glucose levels and prevent hypoglycemia, then most patients with type 1 diabetes should do a minimum of four tests per day. Two tests per day, before breakfast and dinner, usually do not provide enough information to help adjust insulin and diet in patients, even in those taking two injections a day. Patients should test at least four times per day, before breakfast, lunch, dinner, and bedtime. Additional tests before, during, and/or after exercise can help the patient avoid serious hypoglycemia (see Exercise, page 108). Adding a test periodically postmeal and in the middle of the night is particularly important for patients who aim for near-normal blood glucose levels and for any patient during illness or intense physical activity.

Typical testing times for most patients should include prebreakfast (fasting), prelunch, presupper, and bedtime every day. Patients who have asymptomatic nocturnal hypoglycemia should be advised to test their blood glucose at bedtime every night, particularly during very active days. In addition, such patients should test their blood glucose at 2:00–4:00 a.m. four to five times a month. Patients should vary testing times to learn about their blood glucose patterns over the entire day. For patients who are well stabilized on fixed doses of insulin, routine testing (4 times/day) three days a week (including 1 weekend day) may be sufficient to prevent acute hypoglycemic or hyperglycemic crisis but not enough to obtain near-normal glucose control. Patients who are ill (Table 2.7) or whose usual schedule has changed require more frequent monitoring.

Adjusting Insulin Dose

SMBG results are crucial in making appropriate insulin adjustments to optimize glycemic control and prevent hypoglycemia and avoid hyperglycemic crisis. Insulin dose adjustments are covered earlier in this chapter under the section "glycemic targets and insulin adjustments." SMBG results are also used at mealtimes to calculate a correction bolus in addition to the meal bolus needed to cover that meal. Thus, most patients should be encouraged to monitor a minimum of four times a day with additional monitoring at other times (postprandially and nocturnally) to ensure safe and effective therapy.

Pregnant women need to perform SMBG more frequently (6–8 times daily) to adjust insulin doses to obtain glycemic targets and to avoid hypoglycemia. As with other elements of diabetes management, the prescription for SMBG must be individualized.

The value of SMBG is not limited to adjustments in insulin dose. Patients with suspected nocturnal hypoglycemia can check their blood glucose levels at 3:00 a.m. SMBG is a valuable educational tool to help the patient differentiate between symptoms truly arising from hypoglycemia or hyperglycemia and those from other causes.

Common Causes of Errors

Despite the relative simplicity of SMBG, the information is not free of errors. Many of the previous problems with SMBG have been resolved with test strips that do not require wiping and meters with built-in timers. The most common problems now with SMBG, independent of specific methodologies, include the use of an inadequate drop of blood on the strip or a poorly calibrated meter.

These problems stress the need to provide proper patient education and training in SMBG. Finally, some patients report their results inaccurately, perhaps to please their diabetes management team with the right results. The use of meters that automatically store glucose results in an electronic memory may simplify the recording and reporting of SMBG, and these results should be downloaded and analyzed during office visits. Nevertheless, patients should still be encouraged to produce a written record of their test results to detect patterns. Faxing data saves considerable amounts of time and enhances compliance to SMBG and intensive diabetes management.

Successful SMBG

If the goal of SMBG is to improve glycemic control, the diabetes management team should ensure that the patient

- reviews results of glycemic patterns with the diabetes management team
- responds to the results by making appropriate changes in the insulin regimen
- receives the necessary psychosocial support and technical guidance
- monitors frequently, at least before meals and bedtime
- reads and reports tests accurately

To support successful SMBG, there should be mutual efforts to maintain education, motivation, and adherence. Furthermore, it is essential for the diabetes management team to provide feedback by monitoring progress with A1C tests every 3 mo. Results of monitoring should be recorded and reviewed by the health care provider at each office visit. Results can also be phoned, mailed, or faxed between visits. Health care professionals must provide appropriate feedback to the patient based on monitoring results.

GLUCOSE SENSORS

Continuous and intermittent glucose sensing is an adjunct to SMBG and provides a method to optimize glycemic control with prevention of hypoglycemic crisis. Two different methodologies (CGMS by Medtronic MiniMed, GlucoWatch Biographer by Cygnus) have become available, with others in development. Both devices are calibrated by fingerstick SMBG measurements and then sense glucose in the interstitial fluid. Interstitial fluid has been shown to correlate well with blood glucose; however, there is a physiological lag. This lag is usually <5 min in the fasting or premeal state but can be up to 13 min in the postprandial state. The GlucoWatch Biographer has a longer lag time because of its intermittent measuring technique. As a result of the lag time and other factors, these devices are recommended for use as an adjunct to, not a replacement of, SMBG. The glucose trends, rather than the absolute glucose values, obtained from these devices are used to make therapy changes to optimize glucose control. Both devices are discussed below.

Continuous Glucose Monitoring System (CGMS)

The CGMS is a first-generation system used to measure glucose continuously in interstitial fluid for up to 72 h. The system resembles a Holter-style monitor and is prescribed by a physician for retrospective monitoring and interpretation of the readings. To use this system, an electrochemical sensor is inserted by an insertion device into the subcutaneous tissue (usually the abdomen, buttocks, or back) and worn for up to 72 h. The sensor measures glucose every 10 s and provides an average glucose every 5 min for up to 288 readings per day. These readings are collected and stored in a monitor connected by a cable to the sensor. Calibration by fingerstick blood glucose measurements is done at least three times per day with entry of the value into the monitor. Patients are also instructed to keep a food diary and enter event markers for specific behaviors such as eating, insulin administration, exercise, and hypoglycemia symptoms. After wearing the device, the sensor is removed and the monitor is downloaded into a computer for further analysis and evaluation by the health care provider and the patient.

Information obtained from the system can then be used to make recommendations in therapy to optimize glycemic control and prevent hypoglycemia. Multiple patterns and trends in glucose can be identified that were not seen with routine SMBG four times per day. Treatment changes based on CGMS data have been shown to improve glycemic control with less hypoglycemia than SMBG alone. Indications for this system include

- patients with elevated A1C
- patients not at optimal control due to
  - variable unexplained glucose readings
  - severe hypoglycemia or hypoglycemia unawareness

The value of this device for both the patient and the health care provider is that a picture is often worth a thousand words. Patients are more apt to appreciate and understand the need for therapy or behavior changes when presented with a clear graphical representation of their continuous glucose readings.

The next generation of this device will include real-time hypoglycemia and hyperglycemia alerts, followed later by the display of real-time readings. Eventually, closed-loop or semiopen-loop systems will evolve with recommendations to both the patient and an insulin delivery device.

GlucoWatch G2 Biographer

The GlucoWatch G2 Biographer is a glucose-monitoring device that provides automatic, real-time, minimally invasive readings every 10 min for up to 13 h. The device is intended for detecting trends and tracking patterns in glucose levels in adults and children with diabetes both at home and in health care facilities. The device is a supplement to, and does not replace, SMBG.

The system contains a watch monitor with disposable autosensors that last up to 13 h. The device is worn on the forearm where an electric current causes interstitial fluid to enter the autosensor membrane for further analysis every 10 min. The device is calibrated by fingerstick SMBG 2 h after placement of the watch. Each reading represents the glucose level from a time ~15 min earlier. Alerts for both high and low glucose can be set. Approximately 23% of the readings are skipped because of physiological interference from heat, perspiration, and other interfering substances. Because 5% of the readings are inaccurate, any single reading from the device should not be used by itself for treatment change unless an SMBG result is obtained. Interpretation of the results should be based on trends and patterns seen in several sequential readings over time. The watch can store up to 8,500 data points for downloading and further analysis.

Candidates for the GlucoWatch Biographer have not reached their glycemic goals and may have

- hypoglycemia unawareness
- recurrent major hypoglycemia
- frequent hyperglycemia
- A1C >7%

The major adverse effect is skin irritation either from the electrical sensing method or from an allergic reaction to the autosensor adhesive. The irritation usually resolves within a few days to 2 wk, but may result in the inability to wear the device again. Use of an adhesive remover to remove the autosensor minimizes skin irritation. Use of hydrocortisone cream after removal of the autosensor also minimizes irritation. Use of other steroid topical products before placement of the autosensor is under investigation.

KETONE TESTING

The ketone bodies, acetoacetate (AcAc), acetone, and β-hydroxybutyric acid (β-HBA), are catabolic products of free fatty acids. Determinations of ketones in the urine and blood are widely used as adjuncts for both the diagnosis and ongoing monitoring of DKA. Measurements of ketone bodies can be routinely performed both in the office/hospital setting and by patients at home.

Urine ketone testing remains the most commonly used method to detect ketones at home. Most urine methods use reagent strips containing nitroprusside that form a colorimetric reaction on contact with AcAc (and in some strips acetone), resulting in a purple color. Care should be taken not to use out-of-date strips. The strips are manually read as measuring negative, small, moderate, or large ketones. Urine methodologies do not measure β-HBA and are thus not useful in monitoring the response to DKA treatment, because AcAc and acetone may increase as β-HBA falls during successful treatment of DKA.

Testing for ketonuria should be a regular feature of sick-day instructions and should be done every time blood glucose levels are consistently >240 mg/dl (>13.3 mmol/l). The presence of persistent moderate or large amounts of ketones in the urine suggests the possibility of impending or established DKA and should prompt patients to adjust insulin as recommended or seek assistance by calling their health care provider. Note that positive urine ketone readings are found in up to 30% of first morning urine specimens from pregnant woman (with and without diabetes), during starvation, and after hypoglycemia.

Blood ketone testing is also available for home and office/hospital use. Most blood methods measure β-HBA, which is the predominant ketone in DKA. Reference intervals for β-HBA differ among the assay methods, but concentrations <0.5 mmol/l are considered normal, 0.6–1.5 mmol/l indicate the potential for DKA, and >1.5 mmol/l indicate high risk for DKA or that DKA is already present.

Specific measurements of β-HBA in blood can be used by both the patient and health care provider for the diagnosis and monitoring of DKA. Testing for blood ketones is not mandatory by either the patient or the health care provider because the patient can use urine testing to troubleshoot hyperglycemia and the health care provider can use measurements of serum CO_2, anion gap, and pH to diagnose and monitor DKA treatment. However, blood ketone testing is much more specific than urine testing and much quicker and easier than these hospital laboratory methods, and thus has a role in the prevention, diagnosis, and management of DKA.

PHYSICIAN-PERFORMED MONITORING

Because blood glucose levels can fluctuate widely in type 1 diabetes, sporadic testing in the physician's office is not sufficient as the sole means of monitoring. Intermittent testing does not reliably predict glucose levels at other times or the level of chronic glycemic control. Laboratory glucose determinations by a calibrated meter or approved instrument should be performed at each office visit to validate the accuracy of patient-performed monitoring and meter accuracy.

Glycated Hemoglobin (A1C test)

The introduction of the A1C assay has revolutionized the ability to follow glucose control over time. When hemoglobin and other proteins are exposed to glucose, the glucose becomes attached to the protein in a slow, nonenzymatic, and concentration-dependent fashion. The concentration of glycated hemoglobin best reflects the mean blood glucose concentration over the preceding 6–10 wk.

This measurement is performed on a single tube of blood or with a fingerstick capillary sample, and when correctly performed by a reliable laboratory or certified kit, the test is unaffected by acute changes in blood glucose; therefore, the test can be performed at any time during the day.

Assay methods. HbA_{1c} has become the preferred method for assessing glycemic control. In referring to this test, the term "A1C test" has been recommended. A1C can be assayed with several methods that measure different components of the glycated product (e.g., total A1C). Depending on the method used, actual test results, including normal ranges, will vary, and results from different laboratories in the past could not be directly compared. As a result, assay methods have been encouraged to standardize A1C determinations to DCCT values and obtain certification by the National Glycohemoglobin Standardization Program (NGSP). However, certain medical conditions, e.g., hemoglobinopathies, polycythemias, and anemias, may affect the results of some methods. Radioimmunoassay and affinity chromatography methods are usually not affected by hemoglobinopathies.

Utility. A properly performed A1C test provides the best available index of chronic glucose levels. Other glycated protein molecules can be measured for this purpose (e.g., glycated albumin or fructosamine), but their role in clinical practice is less well established.

A1C testing is invaluable in identifying patients who have relatively high, average, or near-normal levels of chronic glucose control. Discrepancies between the A1C level and the results of SMBG may indicate that the latter is either inaccurately performed or fabricated. A less likely possibility is that the patient has some form of hemoglobinopathy that is interfering with the A1C assay: sickle hemoglobin spuriously lowers results, whereas HbF may spuriously elevate glycated hemoglobin in some assays.

The measurement of A1C allows physician and patient to set objective goals for therapy and to measure the efficacy of changes in therapy. The usual frequency for performing this assay in type 1 diabetes should be four times per year.

A1C testing at the time of the patient's visit with immediate results at that time is available by multiple, NGSP-certified, assays and kits. Such testing allows the patient and physician to discuss the results at that visit and make immediate changes in treatment if needed to optimize glycemic control. Such point-of-care testing has resulted in a 0.5– to 1–percentage point drop in the A1C value. A1C testing by home NGSP-certified kits has also recently been approved. Value of such testing remains to be determined.

CONCLUSION

The appropriate application of SMBG techniques provides the patient with type 1 diabetes the opportunity to adjust therapy safely and effectively. The type and frequency of monitoring must be individualized and will be dictated primarily by the patient's lifestyle and the intensity of insulin therapy. A1C testing provides an objective index of long-term glucose levels and can be used to determine efficacy of treatment.

BIBLIOGRAPHY

American Diabetes Association: Tests of glycemia in diabetes (Position Statement). *Diabetes Care* 26 (Suppl. 1):S106–S108, 2003

Bode BW, Gross TM, Thornton KR, Mastrototaro JJ: Continuous glucose monitoring to adjust diabetes therapy improves glycosylated hemoglobin: a pilot study. *Diabetes Res Clin Pract* 46:183–190, 1999

Bode BW, Sabbah H, Davidson PC: What's ahead in glucose monitoring? *Postgrad Med* 109:41–44, 2001

Boland EA, Delucia M, Brandt CA, Grey MJ, Tamborlane WV: Limitations of conventional methods of self blood glucose monitoring: lessons learned from three days of continuous glucose monitoring (CGMS) in pediatric patients with type 1 diabetes. *Diabetes* 49 (Suppl. 1):397, 2000

Chase HP, Kim LM, Owen SL, MacKenzie TA, Klingensmith GJ, Murtfeldt R, Garg SK: Continuous subcutaneous glucose monitoring in children with type 1 diabetes. *Pediatrics* 107:222–226, 2001

Cheyne EH, Cavan DA, Kerr D: Performance of a continuous glucose monitoring system during controlled hypoglycaemia in healthy volunteers. *Diabetes Technol Ther* 4:607–613, 2002

Eastman RC, Chase HP, Buckingham B, et al.: Use of the GlucoWatch Biographer in children and adolescents with diabetes. *Pediatric Diabetes* 3:127–134, 2002

Jungheim K, Koschinsky T: Risky delay of hypoglycemia detection by glucose monitoring at the arm. *Diabetes Care* 24:1303–1304, 2001

Kerr D, Cheyne EH, Weiss M, Ryder J, Cavan DA: Accuracy of MiniMed continuous glucose monitoring system during hypoglycaemia. *Diabetology* 44 (Suppl. 1):A239, 2001

Mastrototaro J: The MiniMed continuous glucose monitoring system (CGMS). *J Pediatr Endocrinol Metab* 12:751–758, 1999

Nathan DM, Singer DE, Hurxthal K, Goodson JD: The clinical information value of the glycosylated hemoglobin assay. *N Engl J Med* 310:341–46, 1984

Pitzer K, Desai S, Dunn T, Edelman S, Jayalakshmi Y, Kennedy J, Tamada JA, Potts RO: Detection of hypoglycemia with the GlucoWatch Biographer. *Diabetes Care* 24:881–885, 2001

Sacks DB, Bruns DE, Goldstein DE, Maclaren NK, McDonald JM, Parrott M: Guidelines and recommendations for laboratory analysis in the diagnosis and management of diabetes mellitus. *Clin Chem* 48:436–472, 2002

Salardi S, Zucchini S, Santoni R, Ragni L, Gualandi S, Cicognani A, Cacciari E: The glucose area under the profiles obtained with continuous glucose monitoring system relationships with HbA1c in pediatric type 1 diabetic patients. *Diabetes Care* 25:1840–1844, 2002

Schiaffini R, Ciampalini P, Fierabracci A, Spera S, Borrelli P, Bottazzo G, Crinò A: The Continuous Glucose Monitoring System (CGMS) in type 1 diabetic children is the way to reduce hypoglycemic risk. *Diabetes Metab Res Rev* 18:324–329, 2002

Schiffrin A, Belmonte M: Multiple daily self-glucose monitoring: its essential role in long-term glucose control in insulin-dependent diabetic patients treated with pump and multiple subcutaneous injections. *Diabetes Care* 5:479–484, 1982

Schiffrin A, Suissa S: Predicting nocturnal hypoglycemia in patients with type 1 diabetes treated with continuous subcutaneous insulin infusion. *Am J Med* 82:1127–1132, 1987

Shalwitz RA, Farkas-Hirsch R, White NH, Santiago JV: Prevalence and consequences of nocturnal hypoglycemia among conventionally treated children with diabetes mellitus. *J Pediatr* 116:685–89, 1990

Speiser PW: Continuous glucose monitoring in managing diabetes in children. *Diabetes Metab Res Rev* 18:330–331, 2002

Tierney MJ, Tamada JA, Potts RO, Eastman RC, Pitzer K, Ackerman NR, Fermi SJ: The GlucoWatch Biographer: a frequent, automatic and non-invasive glucose monitor. *Ann Med* 32:632–641, 2000

NUTRITION

The effectiveness of medical nutrition therapy (MNT) in the medical management of type 1 diabetes is well established. MNT includes a comprehensive assessment of the patient's nutritional status, diabetes and health status, lifestyle, support systems, and willingness and ability to make changes or initiate new behaviors. MNT is implemented in a nutrition care plan based on individual goals negotiated with the patient and monitoring and evaluation of goal-directed activities. Success and satisfaction are measured by goal achievement and improved metabolic and other health outcomes.

Managing food is one of the most challenging aspects of diabetes self-management and requires knowledge, time, effort, and commitment from those involved. Although there are many other variables beside food that affect blood glucose levels, physicians and other diabetes management care team members often attribute poor glycemic control to a lack of dietary adherence. In the worst-case scenario, the patient is labeled a "diet failure." In the best-case scenario, all team members are knowledgeable about nutrition therapy and supportive of the person with diabetes who is struggling to make lifestyle changes. Because of the complexity of nutrition issues, it is recommended that a registered dietitian, knowledgeable and skilled in implementing diabetes MNT, be the team member providing MNT. Patients with type 1 diabetes should be referred when diagnosed, then routinely consult with a registered dietitian as part of the continuing medical care of their diabetes. Follow-up may be appropriate every 3–6 mo for children and every 6–12 mo for adults.

NUTRITION RECOMMENDATIONS

The American Diabetes Association has published evidence-based nutrition principles and recommendations for the treatment and prevention of diabetes and related complications. These recommendations attempt to translate research data and clinically applicable evidence into nutrition care. The Institute of Medicine's Food and Nutrition Board of the National Institutes of Health (NIH) has recently published dietary reference values for the intake of macronutrients. This report covers Dietary Reference Intakes (DRIs) for energy, carbohydrates, fiber, fat, fatty acids, cholesterol, protein, and amino acids. Competing with the science-based recommendations are media and commercially generated nutrition recommendations based on misinformation, opinion, and a desire to sell a product or program. The target audience for these questionable products and practices is often individuals with chronic disease lured by the promise of a quick or easy solution.

The diabetes management team members must not only be knowledgeable about science- or evidence-based recommendations, but must also be aware of the latest health or nutrition fad or product in the marketplace. When applying scientific principles and recommendations, team members will continue to focus on the patient's individual circumstances and preferences. The patient is the central team member and the one who most actively manages his or her diabetes.

The Nutrition Prescription

The "ADA Diet" as a formulated prescription of calorie and macronutrient composition has been replaced by an individualized nutrition prescription based on nutrition assessment and treatment goals. Specific goals of diabetes MNT are to

- attain and maintain optimal metabolic outcomes, including
  - blood glucose levels in the normal range or as close to normal as is safely possible to prevent or reduce the risk for complications of diabetes
  - a lipid and lipoprotein profile that reduces the risk for macrovascular disease
  - blood pressure levels that reduce the risk for vascular disease
- prevent and treat the chronic complications of diabetes; modify nutrient intake and lifestyle as appropriate for prevention and treatment of obesity, dyslipidemia, cardiovascular disease, hypertension, and nephropathy
- improve health through healthy food choices and physical activity
- address individual nutritional needs, taking into consideration personal and cultural preferences and lifestyle while respecting the individual's wishes and willingness to change

Nutrition recommendations advise that macronutrient composition and distribution be individualized to achieve desired metabolic outcomes (Table 3.8).

NUTRITION THERAPY FOR TYPE 1 DIABETES

Nutritional management of type 1 diabetes requires careful attention to the glycemic effect of foods to contain postprandial blood glucose excursions, maximize the effectiveness of exogenous insulin, and minimize hypoglycemia. MNT also must provide for optimal growth and development of the individual and reduce nutrition-related health risks. Although individuals with diabetes have the same

Table 3.8 Nutrition Recommendations: Historical Perspective

Year	Distribution of Calories		
	Carbohydrate (%)	Protein (%)	Fat (%)
Before 1921		Starvation diets	
1921	20	10	70
1950	40	20	40
1971	45	20	35
1986	50–60	12–20	30
1994	A	10–20	A, B
2002	A, C	15–20*	A, B, C, D

A, based on nutrition assessment; B, <10% saturated fat; C, carbohydrate and monounsaturated fatty acids together = 60–70% energy intake; D minimize intake of *trans* fatty acids
*If renal function is normal.

nutritional needs as individuals without diabetes, the amount and type of food and coordination with insulin delivery directly affect blood glucose levels (Fig. 3.5).

Insulin Regimens

Individuals on multiple daily injections (MDI) of insulin or CSII therapy, i.e., insulin pumps, should adjust their premeal short- or rapid-acting insulin based on the total amount of carbohydrate in their meals. Those receiving fixed daily insulin doses should emphasize consistency of daily carbohydrate content at meals and snacks. Along with the type of insulin regimen, the nutrition care plan addresses caloric requirements, macro- and micronutrient intake, the glycemic effect of foods and meal patterns, lifestyle, exercise, overall health status, and patient goals.

Caloric Requirements

Calories should be prescribed to achieve and maintain reasonable body weight. Note that reasonable weight is defined as the weight an individual and health care provider acknowledge as achievable and maintainable, both short and long term. This may not be the same as traditionally defined desirable or ideal body weight. Daily caloric requirements vary depending on age, gender, body size, and activity patterns. Additional calories are needed to promote growth during childhood, adolescence, pregnancy and lactation, and for catabolic illnesses.

The Estimated Energy Requirement (EER) is defined by the Food and Nutrition Board of the Institute of Medicine as "the dietary energy intake that is predicted to maintain energy balance in a healthy individual of a defined age, gender, weight, height, and level of physical activity consistent with good health." The Food and Nutrition Board has published several tables of EER for adults based on body mass index (BMI) and four physical activity levels: sedentary, low active, active, and very active. The board also published gender- and age-based EER tables for infants, children, and adolescents. These tables are available on the Internet from the National Academies Press web site (see Resources for Professionals). Several other methods for estimating caloric requirements are available, including the Harris-Benedict or World Health Organization equations, which compute calories for basal or resting energy expenditure (REE) and then

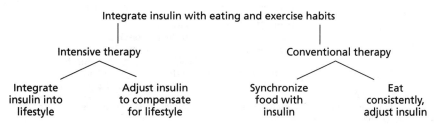

Figure 3.5 Medical nutrition therapy for type 1 diabetes.

add activity calories to the basal requirement. Simple methods for routine use are outlined in Table 3.9. Accurate records of food intake offer another means for estimating energy requirements and provide useful information on food preferences and eating patterns. Adjustments in caloric intake will need to be made to promote growth, weight gain, weight loss, or weight maintenance. In addition to meeting energy requirements, the caloric prescription promotes a consistency in daily food intake that is helpful in managing type 1 diabetes.

Macronutrients

In general, recommendations for the macronutrient composition of the meal plan for diabetes correspond to guidelines for healthy eating for all Americans. The composition and distribution will be guided by the individual's needs and preferences.

Carbohydrate

The primary role of carbohydrates (sugars and starches) is to provide energy to cells in the body. The RDA for carbohydrate is set at 130 g/day for adults and children and is based on the average minimum amount of glucose utilized by the brain.

Carbohydrate Classification

Carbohydrates are divided into categories based on the number of sugar units. The categories of greatest interest in diabetes care and education are sugars (monosaccharides, disaccharides, and polyols), and polysaccharides (starches and nonstarch polysaccharides [fiber]) (Table 3.10). The terms *complex carbohydrates*

Table 3.9 Estimating Adult Daily Energy Needs

Adults

Basal calories	20–25 kcal/kg desirable body wt	
	25–35 kcal/kg for catabolic illness	
Add calories for activity	If sedentary	30% more calories
	If moderately active	50% more calories
	If strenuously active	100% more calories
Adjustments	Add 500 kcal/day to gain 1 lb/wk	
	Subtract 500 kcal/day to lose 1 lb/wk	
	Pregnancy: add 340 kcal/day during 2nd trimester,	
	452 kcal/day during 3rd trimester*	
	Lactation: add 500 kcal/day during 1st 6 mo,	
	400 kcal/day during 2nd 6 mo*	

Adapted from Joyce M: Issues in prescribing calories. In *Handbook of Diabetes Medical Nutrition Therapy*, p. 368.
*Food and Nutrition Board Institute of Medicine: *Dietary Reference Intakes for Energy, Carbohydrate, Fiber, Fat, Fatty Acids, Cholesterol, Protein, and Amino Acids (Macronutrients)*. See Bibliography.

Table 3.10 Classification of Carbohydrates

Class	Subgroup	Components
Sugars	Monosaccharides	Glucose, galactose, fructose
	Disaccharides	Sucrose, lactose
	Polyols	Sorbitol, mannitol, xylitol
Polysaccharides	Starch	Amylose, amylopectin, modified starches
	Nonstarch polysaccharides (fiber)	Cellulose, hemicellulose, pectins, hydrocolloids

and *simple sugars* are no longer used. Intrinsic sugars are sugars that are present within the cell walls of plants (naturally occurring), whereas extrinsic sugars are those which are typically added to foods. Added sugars are defined as sugars and syrups that are added to foods during production and do not include naturally occurring sugars such as lactose in milk or fructose in fruits. Foods and beverages with a high added sugar content include soft drinks, cookies, cakes, pastries, and candy. These foods and beverages have lower micronutrient densities compared to those that are major sources of naturally occurring sugars. Current US food labels do not distinguish between sugars naturally present in foods and added sugars. Traditionally, sugars, particularly sucrose, have been restricted in diets for individuals with diabetes. However, studies show that this restriction is not warranted metabolically. The USDA Food Guide Pyramid guidelines allow up to 25% of calories to come from added sugars. However, carbohydrates providing essential nutrients should receive first priority in food choices before selecting foods and beverages high in added sugars and low in nutrient density.

Healthy carbohydrates. Foods containing carbohydrate from whole grains, fruits, vegetables, and low-fat milk are important sources of vitamins, minerals, phytochemicals, and fiber. Therefore, a liberal intake of these nutrient-dense carbohydrates is recommended for Americans, including those with diabetes. Healthy eating programs such as the Five a Day program and the Dietary Approaches to Stop Hypertension (DASH) diet encourage increased intake of fruits and vegetables, whole grains, and low-fat milk.

Glycemic effect of carbohydrate. The American Diabetes Association's position states that the total amount of carbohydrate in meals and snacks is a better predictor of glycemic response than the source (starch or sugar) or type (glycemic index). Individuals using MDI or CSII therapy should adjust premeal insulin doses based on the total carbohydrate content of the meal. Those on fixed doses of insulin should be consistent with their carbohydrate intake. There is widespread interest and controversy surrounding the concepts of glycemic index and glycemic load. See Figures 3.6 and 3.7 for definitions.

Glycemic index. Glycemic index (GI) is a concept and meal planning approach based on published tables ranking carbohydrate foods according to

"The glycemic index is a classification proposed to quantify the relative blood glucose response to carbohydrate-containing foods. It is defined as the area under the curve for the increase in blood glucose after the ingestion of a set amount of carbohydrate in an individual food (e.g., 50 g) in the 2-h postingestion period as compared with ingestion of the same amount of carbohydrate from a reference food (white bread or glucose) tested in the same individual under the same conditions using the initial blood glucose concentration as a baseline."

Figure 3.6 Glycemic Index: Institute of Medicine's Food and Nutrition Board definition.

glycemic response (Fig. 3.6). The tables propose that, per gram of carbohydrate, foods with a high GI produce a higher peak in postprandial blood glucose and a greater overall glucose response during the first 2–3 h after consumption than do foods with a low GI. *The International Table of Glycemic Index and Glycemic Load Values: 2002* contains 1,300 data entries representing 750 different types of foods tested. Study subjects included "healthy" volunteers and those with type 1 or type 2 diabetes. Type 1 diabetes subjects participated in the study of 17% of the foods included in the table.

The concept of GI seemed straightforward when it was first introduced as a research tool in the 1980s, but the use of GI in preventing and treating disease has created much controversy. Proponents of GI support its role in treating and preventing chronic disease, including diabetes, obesity, coronary heart disease, and cancer. Critics of GI point out flaws in epidemiologic studies cited in support of GI as a public health tool. Additional concerns are related to the utility of the tables as a tool for nutritional management. Within each food category there is wide variability; values can vary as much as fivefold, depending on the food form, study setting, and other factors. In earlier studies, cooked carrots received a GI rating of 92 ±20, whereas in more recent studies, they are rated at 32 ±5. Many factors affect the glycemic response, including variation in the food and its preparation and the circumstances under which it is ingested (Table 3.11). Additionally, variability within and between subjects is large.

Glycemic load. The portion sizes for many of the foods studied for GI were not realistic or usual. To obtain 50 g carbohydrate from carrots, almost five cups

"Thus, the GL of a typical serving of food is the product of the amount of available carbohydrate in that serving and the GI of the food." The GL values in the tables were calculated "by multiplying the amount of carbohydrate contained in a specified serving size of the food by the GI value of that food (with the use of glucose as the reference food), which was then divided by 100." Because portion sizes vary from country to country, researchers and health professionals are advised to calculate their own GL data by using appropriate serving sizes and carbohydrate composition data.

Figure 3.7 Glycemic Load: International Table of Glycemic Index and Glycemic Load Values: 2002 definition.

Table 3.11 Factors Affecting the Rate of Digestibility and Glycemic Response

Factors inherent in a food	Grain, particle size
	Amylose-amylopectin (starch) ratio
	Fiber content
	Enzyme inhibitors
	Physical interaction with fat or protein within a food
	Degree of ripeness in fruit
Factors related to preparation	State of hydration
	Raw vs. cooked
	Amount of food processing
Factors related to consumption	Addition of protein, fat, other foods
	Acidity of a meal
	Preceding meal
	Time of day
	Palatability
	Duration of the meal
	Rate of gastric emptying

of cooked carrots would need to be ingested. The concept of glycemic load (GL) was introduced to take into account the amount of carbohydrate in a *usual* serving of a particular food. The GL is calculated using the average GI of the particular food, multiplied by the grams of carbohydrate available in a typical serving of that food (Fig. 3.7). GL has been calculated for the foods listed in the *International Table*. Concerns about GL are based on the use of imprecise values multiplied to give yet another imprecise number. To use GI, or GL, as a meal-planning tool, one would select foods with low or medium GI versus those with a high GI or, if consuming high-GI foods, also select low-GI foods for balance. The assumption is that the higher the GI or GL, the greater the expected elevation in blood glucose and insulin requirements.

Using GI for meal planning. The American Diabetes Association position is that GI adds another level of complexity to meal planning without scientific evidence to recommend its use as a primary strategy. People with type 1 diabetes may find value in identifying foods and circumstances to determine their own personal GI of preferred and frequently used foods and meals. Based on their unique response, they can develop strategies to adjust meal-related insulin accordingly. The starting point is to match premeal insulin doses to the total carbohydrate content of the meal.

Resistant starch. There are no published long-term studies proving benefit from use of resistant starch in subjects with diabetes.

Nutritive Sweeteners

Sucrose. Sucrose restriction in the diet for diabetes cannot be justified on the basis of its glycemic effect. Sucrose can be included in diets of people with diabetes by making appropriate substitutions for other carbohydrate sources to maintain consistent carbohydrate intake. If the sucrose-containing food is added as an extra, it can be covered with additional short- or rapid-acting insulin. Consider the potential for a decrease in nutrient value and an increase in fat intake and calories that often accompanies sucrose-containing foods.

Fructose. Fructose has a low glycemic effect, which suggests that it could be the sweetener of choice for individuals with diabetes. Large amounts of fructose, however, can have an adverse effect on blood lipids. Many products are sweetened with high-fructose corn syrup, which contains substantial amounts of glucose. Fructose provides 4 cal/g and in general does not offer strong advantages over other sweeteners.

Fruit juice, honey, molasses, corn syrup, and other natural sweeteners require the same considerations as sucrose. They contribute 4 cal/g and need to be counted as carbohydrate in meal planning.

Sugar alcohols. Sugar alcohols (e.g., sorbitol) and hydrogenated starch hydrolysates have less of a glycemic effect than sucrose and may yield less than 4 cal/g. Some individuals report gastric discomfort after eating foods sweetened with these products, and consumption of large quantities can cause diarrhea.

Nonnutritive Sweeteners

Nonnutritive sweeteners available in the United States include saccharin, acesulfame potassium, aspartame, and sucralose. Three additional sweeteners are being evaluated by the FDA: alitame, cyclamate (removed from the market in 1970), and neotame. The FDA determines an acceptable daily intake (ADI) for products it approves that is defined as a safe amount for daily consumption over a lifetime. The ADI includes a 100-fold safety factor and greatly exceeds average consumption levels. All FDA-approved sweeteners can be used by individuals with diabetes, including pregnant women. However, moderation is often recommended.

Fiber

Dietary fiber appears to benefit overall bowel health, including prevention and treatment of constipation and possible prevention of colon cancer. Soluble fiber in large amounts has been shown to be effective in reducing total and LDL cholesterol levels in diabetic and nondiabetic subjects. The beneficial effect of soluble dietary fiber on glycemic control, although intuitively attractive, is difficult to substantiate. An overall benefit to blood glucose control from dietary fiber has not been established and may require large amounts (>50 g fiber) to achieve a significant effect. The Food and Nutrition Board of the NIH, for the first time, has indicated an adequate intake (AI) for fiber (Table 3.12). *The Exchange Lists for Meal Planning*'s starch list "nutrition tips" identify foods that provide 2–6 g fiber per serving.

Protein

Daily requirements. There is no evidence to suggest that the usual intake of protein should be modified if renal function is normal. Protein intakes of 15–20% of calories (~1 g protein/kg) are considered adequate to support health in the general population. Studies suggest that consumption of ≥20% of energy as protein may have detrimental effects on renal function. The RDA for protein is 0.8 g/kg/day for adults, which corresponds to ~10% of calories. Protein requirements for children range from 1.5 g/kg/day for infants to 0.85 g/kg/day for adolescent males through 18 yr of age. Some patients who are interested in strength training and muscle development are advised by trainers, coaches, and others to take large amounts of protein or amino acids, often in powdered form, to build muscle. When patients indicate an interest in strength training activities, diabetes clinicians must be prepared to discuss with them safe amounts of protein intake for their individual kidney function status.

Protein and nephropathy. In patients with diabetic nephropathy, reduction of dietary protein to 0.8–1.0 g/kg/day for people with microalbuminuria and 0.8 g/kg/day for people with overt nephropathy may slow the progression of nephropathy. A recent study comparing plant protein versus animal protein meals in individuals with type 2 diabetes and microalbuminuria found no clear advantage for recommending primarily plant protein.

Protein and insulin requirements. Meal doses of insulin are calculated based on the carbohydrate content of the meal, with the assumption that the basal insulin will cover the protein in the meal. The addition of larger than usual amounts of protein to meals may require a small amount of additional insulin 3–5 h following the meal. Individuals using CSII may use extended delivery of meal bolus insulin for this type of meal. A dual-wave bolus can deliver part of the meal bolus before the meal and the remainder over 2–4 h following the meal.

Table 3.12 Adequate Intake for Total Fiber

	Men	Women
Adults under 50 yr	38 g	25 g
Adults over 50 yr	30 g	21 g

Adapted from Food and Nutrition Board Institute of Medicine: *Dietary, Reference Intakes for Energy, Carbohydrate, Fiber, Fat, Fatty Acids, Cholesterol, Protein, and Amino Acids (Macronutrients)*. See Bibliography.

Fat

The 85–90% of daily calories not allocated to dietary protein are distributed between carbohydrate and fat sources. The National Cholesterol Education Program (NCEP) recommends that adults limit fat intake to <35% of calories, with saturated fat intake restricted to <10% of total calories. Saturated fat is highly atherogenic and has a greater impact on serum cholesterol than does dietary cholesterol. The NCEP recommends that polyunsaturated fat intake not exceed 10% of calories but allows flexibility in the area of monounsaturated fat consumption with a suggested intake of up to 20% of total calories. Dietary cholesterol intake should be <300 mg/day.

These recommendations are appropriate for most individuals with type 1 diabetes because diabetes is an independent risk factor for cardiovascular disease, and plasma lipid levels of individuals with controlled type 1 diabetes are similar to those of the general population of the same age and gender. Foods that contain omega-3 fatty acids have cardioprotective effects; the ADA recommends that people with diabetes eat 2–3 servings per week of foods providing omega-3 polyunsaturated fat, such as fish.

If individuals with type 1 diabetes have hyperlipidemia that is not associated with hyperglycemia, appropriate dietary modifications should be used. If LDL cholesterol levels are ≥100 mg/dl, further restriction of saturated fat to <7% of total calories and dietary cholesterol to <200 mg/day is recommended. *Trans* fats are another LDL-raising fat that should be kept at a low intake.

Alcohol

Most adults with type 1 diabetes may drink alcohol in moderation if they so choose. Exceptions include individuals whose blood glucose is out of control, those attempting weight loss, those with elevated blood triglycerides, and pregnant women. Daily intake should be limited to one drink for women and two drinks for men. One drink is 12 oz beer, 5 oz wine, or 1.5 oz 80-proof distilled spirits. Each drink contains 15 g alcohol.

In addition to the precautions regarding alcohol use that apply to the general public, people with type 1 diabetes risk alcohol-induced hypoglycemia when meals are skipped or delayed or during fasting. Therefore, alcoholic beverages should be added to the meal plan without reducing food intake to balance calories derived from alcohol. However, if the patient is on a weight loss regimen, calories from alcohol (7 cal/g) must be considered. A reduction in fat intake can be used to offset calories consumed in an alcoholic beverage.

Micronutrients

Sodium and hypertension. People differ greatly in their sensitivity to sodium and its effect on blood pressure. Because sodium-sensitive individuals are not easily identified, the intake recommendation goal is no more than 2,400 mg/day. The recommendation for people with mild-to-moderate hypertension is ≤2,400 mg/day sodium, and for individuals with hypertension and nephropathy, it is ≤2,000 mg/day. Sodium intake can be minimized by reducing the use of table salt, processed and convenience foods, and fast foods. The *Exchange Lists for Meal Planning* highlights foods with a sodium content >400 mg/serving. The Nutrition Facts panel on food labels provides useful information by indicating, for a single serving, the amount of sodium in milligrams and the percent of the daily value (the % of 2,400 mg). A consumer may wish to reconsider use of a food containing >25% of the daily value.

Potassium. Individuals taking diuretics may experience a loss of potassium sufficient to warrant supplementation. Potassium restriction may be required if hyperkalemia occurs in patients with renal insufficiency or in those taking angiotensin-converting enzyme inhibitors or angiotensin receptor blockers.

Magnesium. Magnesium deficiency can be easily detected and treated. The deficiency may occur as a result of poorly controlled diabetes and the accompanying urinary loss.

Calcium. The Food and Nutrition Board of the Institute of Medicine has established AIs for calcium based on age (Table 3.13). The values are the same for males and females. Because of enhanced absorption of calcium during pregnancy and lactation, calcium requirements are similar to the nonpregnant and nonlactating state and are based on age.

Vitamin and mineral supplementation. At this time, there is no clear evidence that vitamin and mineral requirements of individuals with type 1 diabetes are different from those of other healthy people. If a nutrition assessment reveals a deficiency, individuals should be counseled on how to adjust food intake to meet these needs. If they are unable to do so, supplements should be recommended. When caloric intake is ≤1,200 cal/day, use of a multivitamin and mineral supplement should be advised. Several conditions may create a deficiency in one or more micronutrients that would warrant supplementation. These include poor diabetes control, use of diuretics, critical care environments, medications that alter micronutrient metabolism, strict vegetarian diets, nutritional intakes that do not meet established RDAs or AIs, pregnancy, and lactation. Pregnancy increases requirements for folate and iron.

Table 3.13 Adequate Intake for Calcium

Age	Adequate Intake (mg/day)
0–6 mo	210
7–12 mo	270
1–3 yr	500
4–8 yr	800
9–18 yr	1,300
19–50 yr	1,000
≥51 yr	1,200

Herbal and botanical supplements. Many people who balk at taking prescription or over-the-counter medications view herbal and botanical products as a safe and natural alternative or adjunct to their diabetes management plan. Very few randomized, clinical trials have examined the safety and efficacy of these products, especially for people with diabetes. Herbal and botanical supplements, sports supplements, and other specialty products represent 32% of the $14 billion of annual sales in the dietary supplement industry. The remaining 48% represent sales of vitamins and minerals. The 1994 Dietary Supplement Health and Education Act (DSHEA) changed the regulation of dietary supplements and associated label claims. DSHEA places the burden of proof of unsafe or adulterated products or of false or misleading labeling on the FDA rather than on the manufacturer. However, DSHEA restricts the FDA in regulation of these products. The Federal Trade Commission regulates the advertising of dietary supplements and has taken action against sponsors of false and misleading information. Until proven otherwise, consumers have no assurance that a product contains what the label says it does or that it is free from harmful contaminants. Some herbal preparations have been found to surreptitiously contain pharmaceutical agents that produce hypoglycemia. Health care providers must know when their patients are using these products, although many patients don't voluntarily share this information. While providing individualized, science-based information, it is also important to be sensitive to the patient's decisions to use products that might be considered questionable. The FDA Center for Food Safety & Applied Nutrition and the NIH Office of Dietary Supplements can provide reliable information about many of these products (see Resources, page 106).

ADDITIONAL NUTRITION CONSIDERATIONS

Sick-Day Management

Individuals with type 1 diabetes must be educated to manage brief periods when they cannot ingest solid foods. They must understand the need to continue insulin therapy and carbohydrate consumption. Fruit juices and sugar-containing soda or gelatin can replace the usual carbohydrate in the meal plan. Frequent intermittent intake of small amounts of these foods and beverages helps to provide fluids and energy and helps to avoid hypoglycemia. Individuals should also be taught the value of ingesting fluids containing sodium and potassium (e.g., vegetable and fruit juices and broths) to help replace electrolytes lost from diarrhea and vomiting. The usual meal plan should be reintroduced gradually (see Table 2.7, page 40).

Growth Years

For infants, children, and adolescents, height and weight data can be plotted on standardized growth grids. The caloric prescription for children with diabetes should include adequate calories for growth and development. Poor diabetes control during the growth years can contribute to failure to attain height potential. During these years, it is helpful to schedule visits with the dietitian every 3–6 mo to adjust calories and other nutrients and to account for changes in food preferences and habits. Parents of infants and young children with diabetes may need frequent nutrition counseling to deal with eating challenges common to children that present particular difficulty when coupled with type 1 diabetes.

Pregnancy

The 2002 RDA for pregnant women sets increased calorie requirements at 340 kcal during the 2nd trimester and 452 kcal during the 3rd trimester. The RDA for protein during pregnancy is 1.1 g/kg or an additional 25 g/day protein. The 1990 National Academy of Sciences recommendations for optimum weight gain for pregnant women are based on prepregnancy BMI (Table 3.14). These guidelines anticipate delivery of babies weighing 3–4 kg at term. The 2000 Food and Nutrition Board publication recommends that, to reduce the risk of neural tube defects for women capable of becoming pregnant, 400 µg folic acid should be taken daily from fortified foods, supplements, or both in addition to consuming food folate from a varied diet. Therefore, prescribing a multivitamin plus up to 400 µg/day folate from preconception through the 1st trimester is recommended. The RDA for iron during pregnancy is 27 mg/day. Assessment of nutritional status and dietary intake should guide prescription of supplements. Because of the additional metabolic stress of diabetes on pregnancy, nutritional guidelines need to be individualized for each pregnant diabetes patient to promote optimal blood glucose levels and appropriate maternal and fetal weight gain.

A plan of three meals and three to four snacks will help patients minimize blood glucose excursions and facilitate tight glycemic control. If there is morning ketosis with normal blood glucose levels, the amount of food in the prebedtime snack can be increased or a snack at 3:00 a.m. considered. In the 1st trimester, hyperemesis may be a problem. A very liberal meal plan allowing the patient to eat whatever is tolerated can be helpful. Insulin dosage should be adjusted to allow for minimum food intake at critical points during the day.

Table 3.14 Recommended Weight Gain for Pregnant Women Based on Prepregnancy BMI

Weight-for-Height Category	Recommended Weight Gain	
	kg	lb
Low (BMI <19.8)	12.5–18	28–40
Normal (BMI 19.8–26)	11.5–16	25–35
High (BMI >26–29)	7.0–11.5	15–25
Obese (BMI >29)	≥7.0	≥15

Adapted from Institute of Medicine: *Nutrition During Pregnancy Part I: Weight Gain.* Washington, DC, National Academy Press, 1990. BMI = wt(kg)/ht(m^2).

Lactation

The protein RDA for lactation is an additional 25 g/day above prepregnancy requirements. Additional EER for lactation is based on a milk energy output of 500 kcal/day in the first 6 mo and 400 kcal/day in the second 6 mo. Many women with diabetes report wide swings in blood glucose levels while they are breast-feeding, which may be related to the amount of milk produced and the frequency of feedings. Continuing the pregnancy meal pattern of three meals and three to four snacks may help prevent hypoglycemia and decrease the need for additional insulin to cover the extra calories.

Obesity Management

People with type 1 diabetes may gain excessive weight for several reasons:

- overinsulinization
- frequent and inappropriate treatment of insulin reactions
- efforts to avoid insulin reactions with the use of extra food
- failure to decrease caloric intake to compensate for decreased urinary caloric loss with improved glucose control
- general overemphasis on food intake

Individuals and parents of children with diabetes should be advised about the consequences of obesity on general health. Individuals with diabetes who are attempting to lose weight should avoid fad diets that promote inappropriate food combinations or omissions and rapid weight loss, because dehydration, fluid and electrolyte imbalances, and starvation ketosis may result. Weight loss programs for individuals with type 1 diabetes must include advice about insulin dose adjust-ment, careful monitoring of diabetes control, and realistic weight loss goals.

Long-term maintenance of weight loss is a challenge. Strategies for successful weight management are emerging from the National Weight Control Registry (NWCR), a prospective study of individuals age ≥18 yr who have successfully maintained a 30-lb weight loss for a minimum of 1 yr. The NWCR, a collabora-tive effort between the University of Colorado Health Sciences Center and the University of Pittsburgh School of Medicine, currently includes nearly 3,000 individuals and offers the opportunity to study the eating and exercise habits of successful weight loss maintainers (www.nwcr.ws). The average registrant was overweight as a child (66%), has a family history of obesity, and has a lifetime average gain and loss of 271 lb. Half followed a formal weight loss program. Addi-tional characteristics of the average registrant include:

- has a resting metabolic rate equal to the rate of a nondieting counterpart in the same weight range
- has lost 60 lb and kept it off for 5 yr
- takes in an average of 1,400 calories/day (macronutrient composition is 56% carbohydrate, 19% protein, and 24% fat)
- expends 400 calories/day in exercise
- walks for exercise (77%)
- eats breakfast everyday

NWCR registrants indicate that weight loss maintenance becomes easier over time. Additional strategies used by these registrants include keeping many health foods in the house (87%), keeping records of food intake or exercise (43%), and buying books or magazines related to nutrition or exercise (74%).

Low-Carbohydrate Diets

Low-carbohydrate diets continue to dominate the popular weight loss press. These plans promise people that they will attain successful weight loss while consuming, in some cases, unlimited amounts of protein and fat and restricting carbohydrates. The lure of this simple approach promising satiety and successful weight loss is irresistible to millions of Americans, including people with diabetes. In addition, people with diabetes soon discover that restricting carbohydrates has what seems to be a beneficial effect on blood glucose levels.

The American Diabetes Association and the American Heart Association have declined to endorse these approaches because they lack scientific support for their safety and efficacy with long-term use. There is no reliable evidence of maintenance of weight loss. Additional concerns include the effects of a high fat, high saturated fat intake on lipids and heart disease risk and the effects of high protein intakes on kidney health. Restricting or omitting carbohydrate foods deprives individuals of many nutrient-dense foods with well-documented health benefits. Diabetes clinicians will encounter patients who have independently decided to follow a low-carbohydrate diet or who have been advised by another health professional to do so. Providing the facts about the pros and cons of these plans in a nonjudgmental way will help to increase the patient's receptivity to a healthier alternative.

Eating Disorders

An increasing number of children, adolescents, and adults in the general population appear to be affected with anorexia nervosa, bulimia, or a combination of the two. Disordered eating in type 1 diabetes is more common than previously thought. Type 1 diabetes complicated by an eating disorder is very difficult to manage because of erratic eating patterns and purging behaviors such as vomiting, laxative abuse, or excessive exercise. A purging behavior unique to type 1 diabetes is self-induced glycosuria, achieved by insulin omission. These destructive behaviors can lead to recurrent diabetic ketoacidosis and early development of long-term complications. Recognition and treatment are critical, along with referral to experienced medical, psychological, and nutrition counselors (see Resources, page 106).

THE PROCESS OF MEDICAL NUTRITION THERAPY

The process of MNT begins with a comprehensive assessment of the patient's diabetes status and nutritional status. Following the assessment, the intervention includes collaboration on setting metabolic and self-care goals determined by patient and dietitian as priorities and a plan for action. Achievement of goals will be monitored by ongoing communication between the patient and dietitian. Follow-up visits will provide opportunities to evaluate progress, identify barriers to success, solve problems, and make necessary changes in the plan of care. Although the dietitian is the primary provider of MNT, this component of diabetes management must be integrated into the care provided by all members of the core team. Coordination of this effort is supported by concise and accurate documentation, communication among team members, and consistency of diabetes and nutrition messages provided to the patient.

Assessment

A comprehensive nutrition assessment (Table 3.15) contains components of the medical evaluation and the education assessment for overall diabetes education needs. Recognizing that the other members of the patient's diabetes care team need similar information should encourage communication among clinicians, collaboration on treatment goals, and consistency of messages provided to the patient.

Goal Setting

Specific goals for MNT are identified through the nutrition assessment. These goals must correspond with the overall treatment goals for the individual and must agree with the patient's personal goals for therapy. Goal setting is often

Table 3.15 Nutrition Assessment

Clinical Data

- Height and weight
- Body frame
- Reasonable weight
- Blood pressure
- Family history
- Laboratory data
- Blood glucose and lipids
- A1C
- Abnormal laboratory findings

Nutrition History

- Usual food intake
- Attitudes toward nutrition and health
- Previous nutrition education and outcomes
- Cultural food practices
- Physical activity
- Allergies and intolerances

Nutrient Intake

- Overall nutritional adequacy
- Caloric intake

- Nutrient distribution
- Type of carbohydrate, protein, and fat
- Use of vitamins, minerals, and herbal and botanical products

Social History

- Daily schedule
- Family relationships
- Friends—social support
- Finances and living environment
- Education—learning style
- Self-efficacy

Diabetes and Health Status

- Duration of diabetes
- Insulin regimen
- Hypoglycemia treatment and history
- Diabetes knowledge and skills
- Complications history and current status
- Other medications
- Smoking
- Alcohol

a negotiation process involving clinicians and the patient. Goals should be realistic and specific.

Nutrition Care Plan

The meal plan for type 1 diabetes is directed by the insulin deficiency that characterizes the condition. Food intake and insulin regimens must be coordinated to accommodate the patient's food preferences and lifestyle while achieving goal glucose levels as closely as is safely possible. Fortunately, SMBG, multidose insulin regimens, MDI, and CSII, support this coordination effort. Specific strategies for nutritional management of type 1 diabetes are to

- integrate insulin therapy with an individual's food and physical activity preferences
- base the food plan on assessment of appetite, preferred foods, and usual eating and exercise habits
- use information from SMBG, insulin, food, and physical activity records to make adjustments in food intake or insulin dose to achieve target glucose levels
- modify caloric and nutrient composition of the food plan as appropriate to achieve metabolic and weight goals and for different stages of the life cycle

The individualized self-management plan should also reflect the patient's lifestyle, exercise patterns, and resources. Important considerations include

- daily schedule (weekday and weekend), travel to and from work or school, during work/school, recreational and social activities
- individual's and family's eating patterns, including usual time and size of meals, where meals are eaten, food preferences, social habits, and cultural customs
- availability of food at home, school, or work and food budget
- facilities and equipment for preparation and storage of food

Evaluation

The effectiveness of the nutrition treatment plan is evaluated by outcomes specifically related to the goals of therapy. Outcomes would include metabolic and behavior change measures.

Practice Guidelines for MNT of Type 1 Diabetes

Practice guidelines offer a systematic approach to disease management designed to increase assurance that desired outcomes will be achieved. Nutrition practice guidelines for type 1 and type 2 diabetes were developed using criteria set forth by the Institute of Medicine. In field tests of the nutrition practice guidelines for type 1 diabetes, practice guideline patients achieved greater reduction in A1C than usual care patients. These guidelines are available from the American Dietetic Association (see Resources, page 106).

PRACTICAL APPROACHES TO NUTRITION COUNSELING

Pattern Management

SMBG, insulin, food, and physical activity records provide patients and clinicians an evaluation mechanism that can be used to closely examine the effectiveness of the treatment regimen and to make adjustments to improve glycemic control. Finding and interpreting blood glucose patterns leads to possible changes in either the amount or timing of insulin, food, or physical activity.

Carbohydrate Counting for Intensive Insulin Therapy

Carbohydrate counting is a meal planning approach that focuses on carbohydrate as the primary nutrient affecting postprandial glycemic response. The DCCT increased interest in carbohydrate counting. Carbohydrate counting can be used at basic or advanced levels depending on the interest and skills of the individual.

Basic carbohydrate counting. Carbohydrate counting can be used at a basic level by patients whose goals include consistency of carbohydrate intake to support improved glycemic control. Patients first learn to estimate how much carbohydrate is in their meals and snacks by becoming familiar with reference amounts of foods similar to the Exchange Lists or other published carbohydrate food lists. Other skills include reading food labels accurately for carbohydrate values and estimating carbohydrate amounts in combination foods such as pizza and in restaurants or other meals away from home. A person must be willing to spend time and effort learning and practicing measuring and weighing foods, reading food labels, and using reference books to develop the skills necessary to accurately estimate carbohydrate amounts in portions usually eaten. Nutrient databases are available on the Internet and as software for loading into personal computers or personal digital assistants (palm pilots).

Advanced carbohydrate counting. Individuals on intensive insulin therapy, either MDI or CSII, can learn to match their premeal insulin to their carbohydrate foods using an individualized insulin-to-carbohydrate ratio. Patients striving for tight glucose control while maintaining flexibility in meals and snacks are candidates for using this counting method.

The insulin-to-carbohydrate ratio is determined for individuals based on records of SMBG, insulin doses, food intake, and physical activity. The ratio is based on the amount of short- or rapid-acting insulin needed to cover a specific amount of carbohydrate to achieve postprandial glucose targets. For example, a patient uses 1 unit rapid-acting insulin for every 10 g carbohydrate eaten to achieve a specific blood glucose target 2 h postprandially. Therefore, this person has an insulin-to-carbohydrate ratio of 1:10, i.e., 1 unit insulin covers 10 g carbohydrate. To adjust insulin for varying amounts of carbohydrate, divide the total grams of carbohydrate to be consumed by the insulin-to-carbohydrate ratio. A meal with 100 g carbohydrate would require 10 units of premeal insulin (100 g divided by 10 = 10 units insulin). Some formulas for calculating insulin-to-carbohydrate ratio include weight and total daily insulin dose as part of the equation (e.g., insulin-to-carbohydrate ratio = 2.8 × [wt in lb] divided by total daily dose; see Optimizing Blood Glucose Control, page 65).

An absolute prerequisite for insulin-to-carbohydrate ratio use is that the patient must already be extremely well versed in carbohydrate counting. Time, effort, and practice are needed to become proficient enough in carbohydrate counting to use it safely and effectively in insulin dose calculation and adjustment. The insulin-to-carbohydrate ratio is only a number, and its effectiveness depends on the patient's ability to accurately estimate carbohydrate amounts that can be covered by insulin. Miscalculation of consumed carbohydrate will result in taking too much or too little insulin.

Individuals using insulin-to-carbohydrate ratios also need to consider other factors that affect glycemic response and be aware that they may need to adjust timing of insulin delivery as well as amount of insulin for specific situations. For example, high-fat meals can delay stomach emptying and may require delivery of a divided dose of insulin, such as part of the dose before and part after the meal. CSII allows delivery of extended boluses that help to accommodate this type of insulin delivery.

Nutrition Self-Management Tools

Meal planning tools, such as the *Basic Carbohydrate Counting, Advanced Carbohydrate Counting*, the *Exchange Lists for Meal Planning*, or its simplified version, *Healthy Food Choices*, can be used to guide patients in implementing their nutrition management plan. These tools are available from the American Diabetes Association and the American Dietetic Association. These associations also offer nutrition education materials on several ethnic and regional food practices. The American Diabetes Association has published a variety of cookbooks and a series of menu guides called *Month of Meals* (see Resources, page 106). A meal planning tool should be selected that is appropriate for the patient's lifestyle, reading level, culture, and intensity of diabetes management.

Staged Nutrition Counseling

Eating habits are not easy to change. For the person with type 1 diabetes, the need to balance food intake and activity, the potential for hypoglycemia, and the psychological stress of managing a chronic disease make changing food habits even more difficult. Nutrition counseling should be provided in stages to allow the patient time to absorb information, try out self-management skills, and test the nutrition plan in daily living. Staged nutrition counseling also provides an opportunity to evaluate the effectiveness of the treatment plan and to make modifications to improve diabetes control. MNT is a lifetime treatment of diabetes. Therefore, nutrition counseling must be included in the ongoing care of the patient with type 1 diabetes.

CONCLUSION

Diabetes MNT is more than mere calculation of a caloric prescription with appropriate macronutrient composition and distribution of foods into meals and snacks. It is a complex process that requires commitment on the part of clinicians and the patient to design an individualized nutrition self-management plan. The effectiveness of MNT is evaluated by success in achieving nutrition-related goals. MNT cannot be limited to the time of diagnosis, but must continue through life with adjustments made for growth and development, changes in lifestyle, diabetes status, and health status, and for advances in the field of diabetes nutritional care.

BIBLIOGRAPHY

American Diabetes Association: Evidence-based nutrition principles and recommendations for treatment and prevention of diabetes and related complications (Position Statement). *Diabetes Care* 26:S51–S61, 2003

Davidson PC, Hebblewhite HR, Bode BW, Steed RD, Welch NS, Greenlee MC, Richardson PL, Johnson J: Statistically based CSII parameters: correction factor, CF (1700 rule), carbohydrate-to-insulin ratio, CIR (2.8 rule), and basal-to-total ratio (Abstract). *Diabetes Technol Ther* 5:237, 2003

Delahanty LM, Halford BN: The role of diet behaviors in achieving improved glycemic control in intensively treated patients in the Diabetes Control and Complications Trial. *Diabetes Care* 16:1453–1458, 1993

DCCT Research Group: Nutrition interventions for intensive therapy in the Diabetes Control and Complications Trial. *J Am Diet Assoc* 93:768–772, 1993

Dietary Supplement Health and Education Act of 1994, Public Law 103-417 (S.784) (1994) (codified at 42 USC 287C-11)

Food and Nutrition Board Institute of Medicine: *Dietary Reference Intakes for Calcium, Phosphorus, Magnesium, Vitamin D and Fluoride.* Washington, DC, National Academy Press, 1999

Food and Nutrition Board Institute of Medicine: *Dietary Reference Intakes for Energy, Carbohydrate, Fiber, Fat, Fatty Acids, Cholesterol, Protein, and Amino Acids (Macronutrients).* Washington, DC, National Academy Press, 2002

Food and Nutrition Board Institute of Medicine: *Dietary Reference Intakes for Thiamin, Riboflavin, Niacin, Vitamin B6, Folate, Vitamin B12, Pantothenic Acid, Biotin, and Choline.* Washington, DC, National Academy Press, 2000

Food and Nutrition Board Institute of Medicine: *Dietary Reference Intakes for Vitamin A, Vitamin K, Arsenic, Boron, Chromium, Copper, Iodine, Iron, Manganese, Molybdenum, Nickel, Silicon, Vanadium, and Zinc.* Washington, DC, National Academy Press, 2002

Foster-Powell K, Holt S, Brand-Miller, JC: International table of glycemic index and glycemic load values. *Am J Clin Nutr* 76:5–56, 2002

Franz MJ, Bantle JP, Beebe CA, Brunzell JD, Chiasson JL, Garg A, Holzmeister LA, Hoogwerf B, Mayer-Davis E, Mooradian AD, Purnell JQ, Wheeler M:

Evidence-based nutrition principles and recommendations for the treatment and prevention of diabetes and related complications (Technical Review). *Diabetes Care* 25:148–198, 2002

Gillespie S, Kulkarni K, Daly A: Using carbohydrate counting in diabetes clinical practice. *J Am Diet Assoc* 98:897–905, 1998

Institute of Medicine: *Nutrition During Pregnancy Part I: Weight Gain.* Washington, DC, National Academy Press, 1990

Jenkins DJA, Kendall CWC, Augustin LSA, Franceschi S, Hamidi M, Marchie A, Jenkins AL, Axelsen M: Glycemic index: overview of implications in health and disease. *Am J Clin Nutr* 76 (Suppl.):266S–273S, 2002

Joint National Committee on the Prevention, Detection, Evaluation, and Treatment of High Blood Pressure: *Sixth Report of the Joint National Committee on the Prevention, Detection, Evaluation, and Treatment of High Blood Pressure.* Washington, DC, National Institutes of Health National Heart Lung and Blood Institute, 1997

Joyce M: Issues in prescribing calories. In *Handbook of Diabetes Medical Nutrition Therapy.* Powers MA, Ed. Gaithersburg, MD, Aspen, 1996, p. 368

Klem ML, Wing RR, Lang W, McGuire MT, Hill JO: Does weight loss maintenance become easier over time? *Obesity Res* 8:438–444, 2000

Kulkarni K, Castle G, Gregory R, Holmes A, Leontos C, Power M, Snetselar L, Splett P, Wylie-Rosett J, for the Diabetes Care and Education Dietetic Practice Group: Nutrition practice guidelines for type 1 diabetes mellitus positively affect dietitian practices and patient outcomes. *J Am Diet Assoc* 98:62–70, 1998

National Cholesterol Education Program Expert Panel on Detection, Evaluation, and Treatment of High Blood Cholesterol in Adults (ATPIII): *Third Report of National Cholesterol Education Program (NCEP) Expert Panel on Detection, Evaluation, and Treatment of High Blood Cholesterol in Adults (ATPIII) Executive Summary.* Washington, DC, National Institutes of Health National Heart Lung and Blood Institute, 2001

National Institutes of Health, National Cancer Institute: *5 a Day for Better Health Program Monograph.* Washington, DC, National Institutes of Health, 2002

Peters AL, Davidson MB: Protein and fat effects on glucose response and insulin requirements in subjects with insulin-dependent diabetes mellitus. *Am J Clin Nutr* 58:555–560, 1993

Pi-Sunyer FX: Glycemic index and disease. *Am J Clin Nutr* 76 (Suppl.):290S–298S, 2002

Polonsky WH: Identifying and treating eating disorders in persons with diabetes. In *Handbook of Diabetes Medical Nutrition Therapy.* Powers MA, Ed. Gaithersburg, MD, Aspen, 1996, p. 585–601

Report of a Joint FAO/WHO Expert Consultation: *Carbohydrates in Human Nutrition.* Rome, Italy, Food and Agriculture Organization of the United Nations and World Health Organization, 1998

Sacks FM, Appel LJ, Moore TJ, Obarzanek E, Vollmer WM, Svetkey LP, Bray GA: Dietary approaches to prevent hypertension: a review of the Dietary Approaches to Stop Hypertension (DASH) study. *Clin Cardiol* 22 (Suppl. 7):III6–10, 1999

Sarubin A: *The Health Professional's Guide to Popular Dietary Supplements.* Chicago, American Dietetic Association, 2000

Toeller M, Buyken A, Heitkamp G, Bramswig S, Mann J, Milne R, Gries FA, Keen H, the EURODIAB IDDM Complications Study: Protein intake and urinary albumin excretion rates in the EURODIAB IDDM Complications Study. *Diabetologia* 40:1219–1226, 1997

USDA (US Department of Agriculture): *The Food Guide Pyramid.* Home and Garden Bulletin No. 252. Washington, DC, USDA, 1996

Wheeler ML, Fineberg SE, Fineberg NS, Gibson RG, Hackward LL: Animal versus plant protein meals in individuals with type 2 diabetes and micro-albuminuria: effects on renal, glycemic, and lipid parameters. *Diabetes Care* 25:1277–1282, 2002

RESOURCES FOR PATIENT EDUCATION

Basic Carbohydrate Counting, Advanced Carbohydrate Counting. Alexandria, VA, American Diabetes Association, and Chicago, American Dietetic Association, 2003

Diabetes Care and Education Practice Group of the American Dietetic Association: *Ethnic and Regional Food Practices: A Series.* Alexandria, VA, American Diabetes Association, and Chicago, American Dietetic Association, various publication dates

Exchange Lists for Meal Planning. Alexandria, VA, American Diabetes Association, and Chicago, American Dietetic Association, 2003

Healthy Food Choices. Alexandria, VA, American Diabetes Association, and Chicago, American Dietetic Association, 2003

Month of Meals series. Alexandria, VA, American Diabetes Association, various publication dates

The First Step in Diabetes Meal Planning. Alexandria, VA, American Diabetes Association, and Chicago, American Dietetic Association, 2003

Warshaw HS, Kulkarni K: *Complete Guide to Carb Counting.* Alexandria, VA, American Diabetes Association, 2001

RESOURCES FOR PROFESSIONALS

American Dietetic Association: *Nutrition Practice Guidelines for Type 1 and Type 2 Diabetes Mellitus*. Chicago, American Dietetic Association, 1998

Diabetes Care and Education Practice Group of the American Dietetic Association: *The American Dietetic Association Guide to Diabetes Medical Nutrition Therapy and Diabetes Education*. Chicago, American Dietetic Association, 2003

Franz MJ, Bantle JP (Eds.): *American Diabetes Association Guide to Medical Nutrition Therapy for Diabetes*. Alexandria, VA, American Diabetes Association, 1999

National Academies Press web site for online review of publications on dietary reference intakes for macronutrients and micronutrients: www.nap.edu

NIH Office of Dietary Supplements web site (with IBIDS—International Bibliographic Information on Dietary Supplements—which contains over 690,000 scientific citations and abstracts about dietary supplements): http://dietary-supplements.info.nih.gov

Powers M (Ed.): *Handbook of Diabetes Medical Nutrition Therapy*. Gaithersburg, MD, Aspen, 1996

Sarubin A: *The Health Professional's Guide to Popular Dietary Supplements*. Chicago, American Dietetic Association, 2000

US Food and Drug Administration, Center for Food Safety and Applied Nutrition Dietary Supplements web site. Look under Program Areas for Dietary Supplements: http://vm.cfsan.fda.gov/list.html

Warshaw HS, Bolderman KM: *Practical Carbohydrate Counting: A How-to-Teach Guide for Health Professionals*. Alexandria, VA, American Diabetes Association, 2001

EXERCISE

In addition to insulin and medical nutrition therapy, exercise plays a key role in diabetes management. Important health benefits of physical activity for individuals with diabetes include a reduction in cardiovascular risk factors, increased sensitivity to insulin, better ability to maintain a healthy weight and level of body fat, and a heightened sense of well-being. Given these health benefits, regular physical activity should be considered an integral part of the treatment plan for individuals with type 1 diabetes.

Because exercise can significantly affect blood glucose levels, it must be carefully integrated into the diabetes management regimen. When individuals with type 1 diabetes are given appropriate guidance and support and attain good self-management skills, they can achieve optimal glycemic control, exercise safely, and achieve desired levels of exercise performance. Children and adolescents can participate fully in gym classes, team sports, and other activities. In the absence of contraindications, all adults should accumulate at least 30 min of moderate daily activity to improve health and reduce risk of chronic disease. Adults with type 1 diabetes should be encouraged to achieve at least this level of daily activity. Individuals with physical limitations should be encouraged to maintain an active lifestyle and offered guidance about safe and appropriate exercise options that will enable them to do so.

Success with any physical activity program is greatly enhanced when exercise goals are appropriately established. Goals must be individualized based on a person's interests, likes and dislikes, unique lifestyle and psychosocial variables, age, general health, level of physical fitness, and prior exercise experience.

GLYCEMIC RESPONSE TO EXERCISE

Exercise requires rapid mobilization and redistribution of metabolic fuels to ensure an adequate energy supply for working muscles. For individuals who do not have diabetes, this complex process is coordinated via neural and hormonal responses that increase production of glucose and free fatty acids (FFAs) and facilitate uptake and utilization of these fuels by working muscle (Table 3.16). Insulin levels fall while counterregulatory hormones rise, so that increased glucose utilization by exercising muscle is matched precisely by increased glucose production by the liver. For individuals with type 1 diabetes, the metabolic adjustments that maintain fuel homeostasis during and after exercise are lacking. The result can be a mismatch between hepatic glucose production and muscle glucose utilization and significant deviation from normal glycemia. The glycemic response to exercise can be variable and is influenced by multiple factors. These include

- overall metabolic control
- circulating insulin level
- plasma glucose at the start of exercise
- timing of exercise in relation to food intake
- glycogen stores
- level of training and fitness
- intensity, duration, time, and type of exercise

Table 3.16 Metabolic Response to Light and Moderate Exercise: Normal vs. Type 1 Diabetes

Normal Response	Response in Type 1 Diabetes
Insulin level decreases ■ ⇧ glucose release from liver ■ ⇧ FFA mobilization ■ restricts use of glucose by nonexercising skeletal muscle	Insulin level fails to change at the onset of exercise ■ insulin excess: muscle glucose uptake exceeds liver glucose production ■ insulin deficiency: liver glucose production exceeds muscle uptake; FFA release and ketone body formation increase ■ adequate insulin level: liver glucose output matches muscle glucose uptake
Counterregulatory hormones increase ■ ⇧ hepatic glucose production and release ■ ⇧ muscle glycogenolysis ■ adipose tissue lipolysis	Counterregulatory hormones generally increase, although response may be blunted in some individuals
Glucose uptake and utilization by working muscle increases	Glucose uptake and utilization by working muscle may or may not increase depending on insulin availability
Precise integration of glucose production and utilization and stable blood glucose levels	Potential mismatch between glucose production and utilization and variable blood glucose levels

Plasma insulin level is a primary determinant of the glycemic response to exercise. In individuals who do not have diabetes, the circulating insulin level normally falls at the onset of light or moderate-intensity exercise. In those with type 1 diabetes, this response is absent, and insulin adjustments need to be made in anticipation of exercise. If circulating insulin levels are too high, a state of relative hyperinsulinemia results, which leads to enhanced muscle glucose uptake, inhibited hepatic glucose production, and potentiation of hypoglycemia. In contrast, if circulating insulin levels are too low, as evidenced by preexercise hyperglycemia and poor metabolic control, an inadequate level of insulin combined with a heightened counterregulatory hormone release associated with exercise can lead to a marked increase in glucose production and FFA mobilization from the liver. When availability of these substrates exceeds muscle uptake, a further worsening of glycemic control and ketosis results.

POTENTIAL BENEFITS OF EXERCISE

Because individuals with type 1 diabetes are at high risk for the development of cardiovascular disease, exercise, through its ability to improve multiple cardiovascular risk factors, offers important health benefits. Regular exercise can improve the lipoprotein profile by lowering VLDL cholesterol and triglycerides and by increasing HDL cholesterol. It also can reduce blood pressure, decrease adiposity, improve cardiac work capacity, decrease platelet adhesiveness, and lower the adrenergic response to stress.

Beyond cardiovascular benefits, participation in regular exercise assists with weight loss and is essential for long-term success with maintaining a healthy weight. It enhances sense of well-being and reduces feelings of stress and anxiety. It improves muscle strength and agility, reduces bone loss, and prevents loss of functional capacity that can occur with aging.

Although exercise increases insulin sensitivity and can lower the requirement for insulin, it has not consistently been shown to lead to improvements in glycemic control in individuals with type 1 diabetes as measured by A1C. However, when exercising individuals learn to self-adjust their management to accommodate physical activity through careful meal planning, frequent SMBG and record keeping, and correct application of insulin-adjustment strategies, they can achieve excellent glycemic control and A1C levels.

POTENTIAL RISKS OF EXERCISE

Although exercise offers many health benefits, it also carries potential risks for those with type 1 diabetes. Both acute complications, hyper- and hypoglycemia, and long-term microvascular and macrovascular complications may be exacerbated by physical activity, especially if an exercise option is contraindicated given existing complications or physical limitations or is incorrectly performed.

Hyperglycemia and Hypoglycemia

Because exercise potentiates the effects of insulin, hypoglycemia may occur during, immediately after, or many hours after a period of physical activity. Hypoglycemia poses a risk to individuals who perform unusually long-duration or strenuous exercise or to those who exercise sporadically without adjusting their usual insulin dose or meal plan. In contrast, hyperglycemia can occur if preexercise metabolic control is poor or if exercise is performed at a very high intensity, anaerobic level (>80% of $VO_{2\,max}$).

Individual glycemic response patterns can differ markedly with exercise. SMBG, careful record keeping, and recognition of glucose patterns with activity are important skills that can enable individuals with type 1 diabetes to understand unique glycemic responses to exercise, enhance their ability to make self-management decisions that support optimal glycemic control, exercise safety, and enhance performance. Frequent SMBG helps with anticipation of the onset of hypo- or hyperglycemia and enables individuals to make decisions about taking corrective actions before either complication becomes severe. When data from monitoring are carefully recorded and analyzed, they can provide a valuable basis for making decisions about adjustments in management for subsequent exercise sessions.

Macrovascular and Microvascular Complications

Although regular participation in physical activity tends to reduce cardiovascular risk factors, the risk of arrhythmias, myocardial ischemia or infarction, and cardiac arrest is transiently elevated during exercise. Because individuals with type 1 diabetes are at high risk for cardiovascular disease, careful evaluation to rule out preexisting disease is advisable before an exercise program is initiated. For those with known or suspected disease, a moderate, safe level of exercise that will minimize risk of negative cardiac events should be prescribed.

Screening for microvascular diabetes complications before initiation of exercise is also advisable. Worsening of complications is possible (Table 3.17) if exercise is not carefully prescribed. As for the general population, exercise can aggravate preexisting joint disease or lead to musculoskeletal injuries.

REDUCING EXERCISE RISKS

Potential exercise risks can be reduced if a thorough medical evaluation that includes screenings for microvascular, macrovascular, and neurologic complications of diabetes precedes initiation of exercise (Table 3.18). Based on findings of this exam, an individualized physical activity program should be carefully planned and supported by an appropriate level of supervision to minimize exercise risks and promote progressive gains in health and fitness.

Precautions and Considerations

Exercise should be prescribed with caution in individuals with previous poor metabolic control, including severe hyperglycemia and ketonuria, frequent hypoglycemia or hypoglycemia unawareness, cardiovascular disease, neuropathy,

Table 3.17 Potential Risks of Exercise with Microvascular Diabetes Complications

Microvascular Complication	Potential Exercise Risk
Proliferative retinopathy	Retinal detachment, vitreous or retinal hemorrhage, blood pressure elevation
Peripheral neuropathy	Loss of protective sensation, soft tissue injury, foot ulcers, injury to bones and joints, infection
Autonomic neuropathy	Reduced heart rate and blood pressure response to exercise, silent ischemia, orthostatic hypotension, impaired counterregulatory response to exercise, hypoglycemia unawareness, impaired body temperature regulation, dehydration, reduced exercise tolerance
Nephropathy	Marked blood pressure elevations with high intensity, which may lead to transient increases in proteinuria/albuminuria

Table 3.18 Preexercise Testing Indications for Exercise Program Greater than Brisk Walking

- Age >40 yr
- Age >35 yr and
  - Type 1 or type 2 diabetes of >10 yr duration
  - Hypertension
  - Cigarette smoking
  - Dyslipidemia
  - Proliferative or preproliferative retinopathy
  - Nephropathy, including microalbuminuria
- Any of the following, regardless of age:
  - Known or suspected coronary artery disease, cerebrovascular disease, and/or peripheral vascular disease
  - Autonomic neuropathy
  - Renal failure

proliferative retinopathy, or nephropathy. Individuals with these complications should be offered guidance about safe exercise options as well as activities that should be avoided (Table 3.19). Some individuals may benefit from initially participating in a supervised exercise program. Performance of frequent SMBG before, during, and after exercise should be encouraged.

Participation in a cardiac rehabilitation program may benefit individuals with known cardiovascular disease. For these individuals, the exercise prescription should be based on results of a graded exercise test. Special precautions and

Table 3.19 Exercise Options with Diabetes Complications

Diabetes Complication	Best Exercise Options	Inadvisable Exercise Options
Proliferative retinopathy	Low impact activities like walking, swimming, low-impact aerobics, stationary cycling	Pounding, jarring, or "head-low" activities, high impact sports, heavy lifting, breath-holding and Valsalva-like maneuvers
Insensitive feet/peripheral vascular insufficiency	Non-weight-bearing activities like cycling, swimming, arm chair exercises, light weight lifting, yoga, tai chi	Repetitive weight-bearing or high-impact activities like prolonged walking or jogging
Nephropathy	Light to moderate daily activities, low-intensity aerobic activity, light weight lifting	Heavy lifting or intensive exercise that results in blood pressure increase
Hypertension	Dynamic exercises that primarily use large, lower-extremity muscle groups	Heavy lifting and Valsalva-like maneuvers

monitoring are warranted for those who have hypertension or thyroid disease and for anyone who is taking cardiac or blood pressure medications that can mask hypoglycemia, alter heart rate response to exercise, or influence cardiac work capacity (e.g., β-blockers).

EXERCISE PRESCRIPTION

Before initiating exercise, all individuals should be given specific guidance about appropriate exercise options, exercise goal setting, methods for self-monitoring exercise performance, strategies for maintaining optimal glycemic control, and exercise safety precautions (Table 3.20).

The purpose of an exercise prescription is to offer specific exercise recommendations that will safely and successfully guide an individual toward achieving a level of physical activity that will improve health, fitness, functional capacity, and quality of life. Individualization is the key to success of any exercise program. Unique lifestyle variables, likes and dislikes regarding exercise options, stage of readiness to make necessary lifestyle changes, age, prior exercise experience, and level of fitness should all be considered.

Table 3.20 Exercise Safety Guidelines

General

- Carry a medical identification card and wear an identification bracelet, necklace, or tag that alerts others that individual has diabetes
- Exercise with an informed partner
- Measure preexercise blood glucose and take appropriate action:
  - If <100 mg/dl: eat a carbohydrate-containing snack before exercising
  - If >250 mg/dl: test for ketones and troubleshoot reason for hyperglycemia; if ketones present, delay exercising until ketones are negative
- Frequently consume fluids before, during, and after exercise to prevent dehydration
- Do visual and tactile inspections of feet before and after exercise
- Wear footwear and clothing that is appropriate for the activity you plan to do and for the exercise climate
- Avoid exercising in extreme heat, humidity, or cold

To Prevent Hypoglycemia

- Perform SMBG periodically during prolonged exercise; monitor more frequently postexercise
- Be alert for signs of hypoglycemia during and several hours after an exercise session
- Avoid exercising during peak insulin action
- Administer insulin away from working limbs if exercise is to be initiated within 30 min of an insulin injection
- Consider reducing the dose of insulin that will be acting during a period of exercise
- Have immediate access to a source of readily absorbable carbohydrate (such as glucose tablets) to treat hypoglycemia

Recommendations regarding frequency, intensity, duration, and type of exercise should similarly be individualized. The most precise exercise prescriptions are based on exercise testing that determines heart rate and blood pressure response to exercise and aerobic capacity ($VO_{2\,max}$).

An aerobic conditioning program is desirable for most individuals with diabetes. In addition, all people can benefit from informally increasing daily lifestyle activities (e.g., walking and climbing stairs). The very unfit person may benefit from beginning with a lifestyle activity program before progressing to structured, aerobic exercise.

Whenever possible, an exercise contract that guides an individual toward achieving exercise goals should be established. Goals should be established collaboratively with input from the exercising individual. The person's progress toward achieving goals should regularly be assessed and the exercise plan adjusted as needed. Specific recommendations that are established with active involvement and input from the individual with diabetes are most likely to lead to successful exercise outcomes.

AEROBIC TRAINING

Individuals who are interested and physically able should be encouraged to participate in aerobic activity. Aerobic training, which uses large muscle groups repetitively and continuously for an extended time, promotes optimal improvements in cardiorespiratory fitness, body composition, functional capacity, and overall health when it is consistently done at a level that accrues an energy expenditure of 1,000–2,000 calories per wk. Generally, aerobic activity should be performed

- 20–60 min per session
- 150 min/wk
- at an intensity of 55–79% of maximum heart rate (40–74% of VO_2R maximal oxygen uptake reserve [VO_2R] or heart rate reserve [HRR]), or rating of perceived exertion (RPE) of 12-13-14 "somewhat hard" level of effort (Fig. 3.9); a lower intensity of 55–65% of maximum heart rate (40–50% of VO_2R or HRR), and RPE of 12 is appropriate for those who are unfit (Table 3.21)

Participation in aerobic exercise is safest and most effective if individuals monitor exercise intensity to ensure that they are working in an appropriate "target zone" or level of effort. Three methods that can be used to monitor exercise intensity are heart rate or pulse count monitoring, RPE, and the "talk test" (Tables 3.21 and 3.22). Individuals with known coronary artery disease should be informed about symptoms of myocardial ischemia. Exercise-related chest pain or discomfort, excessive shortness of breath, lightheadedness, or nausea are all indicators that an individual should immediately stop an activity. Any discomfort or worrisome symptoms associated with exercise should be reported to an individual's physician.

Table 3.21 Methods of Determining and Monitoring Exercise Intensity with Exercise

Target Heart Rate	Rating of Perceived Exertion	"Talk Test"
Monitor 10-s pulse count by palpating carotid or radial pulse or use heart rate monitor	Determine perception of effort required or level of difficulty associated with exercising at a given workload	Assess ability to talk or carry on a conversation while exercising as an indicator of staying within/not exceeding an aerobic training level
Target heart rate: 55–79% of HR_{max} or 40–74% VO_2R or HRR*	Target: rating of perceived exertion of 12-13-14 "somewhat hard" level of effort (Table 3.22)	Target: Maintaining ability to talk during an exercise session; avoid extreme shortness of breath

*HR_{max} = 220 – age (or maximal heart rate achieved on exercise stress test)
VO_2R = $VO_{2\,max}$ – resting VO_2 (maximal oxygen uptake reserve; can be calculated if $VO_{2\,max}$ is measured during exercise stress test). HRR = $(HR_{max} – HR_{rest}) + HR_{rest}$ (heart rate reserve; formula accounts for true resting as well as maximal heart rate)

Each session of aerobic exercise should include a 5- to 10-min warm-up and a 5- to 10-min cool-down period. The warm-up should include light general muscle movement, e.g., slow walking or stationary cycling, followed by stretching. The warm-up should be followed by the more vigorous aerobic training period during which the exercise "target zone" should be achieved. At the end of an exercise session, a cool-down period should include light general muscle movement and stretching. Calisthenics or other light resistance activities can be incorporated into the cool down. The heart rate should approach a resting level (<100 beats/min) before the cool down is completed.

When prescribing exercise, it is important to start each individual at a level that can reasonably be achieved. This may require that an individual who is very deconditioned begin by doing short, 5- to 10-min exercise sessions two to three times per day. The duration of each session can gradually be increased as a person becomes more fit. As the duration of each exercise session increases, the number of daily sessions can be reduced. It is important not to overlook the considerable health benefits that can be gained even if exercise is performed at an intensity below an optimal target range for improving cardiorespiratory fitness. Promoting all types of physical activity, even forms that require a low-to-moderate level of effort, is important. For individuals who dislike vigorous exercise, a physical activity program that focuses on weekly energy expenditure rather than on intensity of exercise may support improved adherence and better exercise outcomes.

Resistance exercises such as weight lifting or calisthenics can improve body composition, increase muscle strength and endurance, improve flexibility, increase

Table 3.22 Borg Rating of Perceived Exertion (RPE) Scale

RPE	Perceived Effort
6	
7	Very, very light
8	
9	Very light
10	
11	Fairly light
12	
13	Somewhat hard
14	
15	Hard
16	
17	Very hard
18	
19	Very, very hard
20	

From Borg GA: Physiological bases of perceived exertion. *Med Sci Sports Exerc* 14:377– 387,1982.

insulin sensitivity and glucose tolerance, and decrease cardiovascular risk factors. Individuals who are interested in resistance exercise should be carefully screened for diabetes complications so that a program can be safely adapted to minimize risk of aggravating existing complications. All individuals should be taught proper technique at the onset of a training program to minimize the risk of injury.

If a diabetes clinician does not feel knowledgeable enough about principles of exercise to prescribe and supervise an aerobic exercise program, a referral should be made. Hospital-based cardiac rehabilitation or wellness programs, YMCA programs, and programs offered through college and university physical education departments can be excellent and appropriate options for exercise referral. A well-qualified exercise physiologist or exercise specialist who has clinical experience and is knowledgeable about diabetes can also be a valuable resource.

STRATEGIES FOR MAINTAINING OPTIMAL GLYCEMIC CONTROL WITH EXERCISE

Based on results of SMBG, record keeping, and identification of exercise-related blood glucose patterns, individuals with type 1 diabetes can learn to make adjustments in their diabetes management to maintain optimal glycemic control with exercise. Adjustments can be made in the meal plan, insulin dosage, or both in combination. Diligence with glucose monitoring (before, during, and after exercise), careful record keeping, and well-informed interpretation of blood glucose response patterns are crucial for success with making sound exercise-related adjustment decisions.

Adjusting Carbohydrate Intake

The decision to adjust carbohydrate intake for exercise should be based on a number of factors. These include preexercise blood glucose level, planned exercise intensity and duration, the time of day of the planned activity and time in relation to previous food intake, an individual's level of training, and previous glycemic response to exercise. Additional carbohydrate may be necessary to prevent hypoglycemia, treat hypoglycemia if it occurs, or fuel muscle and delay fatigue during periods of prolonged activity.

When an activity session is of short duration or is unplanned, consuming additional carbohydrate is useful. For moderate activity lasting <30 min, insulin adjustment is rarely necessary, but a small snack that provides ~15 g carbohydrate may be needed. Consuming additional carbohydrate is certainly indicated if the preexercise blood glucose is <100 mg/dl (<5.6 mmol/l). During periods of prolonged or intense exercise when energy expenditure is high, additional carbohydrate is often necessary. Intake of 15 g carbohydrate every 30–60 min of activity is a general, safe starting guideline. Extra carbohydrate may also be needed in the postexercise period when insulin sensitivity is increased and glycogen storage is enhanced. Intake of additional carbohydrate at this time can reduce risk of hypoglycemia and enhance glycogen storage. For individuals who exercise in the late afternoon or evening, it is particularly important to be alert to the possibility of nocturnal hypoglycemia and adjust the evening snack as needed to prevent its occurrence.

The rigid recommendation to consume extra carbohydrate based only on the planned intensity and duration of exercise and without regard to the glycemic level at the start of exercise, previous metabolic response to exercise, and insulin therapy is no longer appropriate. Such an approach can easily neutralize the beneficial blood glucose–lowering effect and energy deficit that results from exercise. The amount of carbohydrate required to prevent hypoglycemia and optimize exercise performance must be determined on an individual basis and can vary with each exercise situation.

Adjusting Insulin

The increasing use of intensive insulin therapy has provided individuals with type 1 diabetes with great flexibility and the ability to make precise insulin adjustments for various activities. In certain exercise situations, it may be necessary to reduce the insulin dosage to prevent hypoglycemia.

A reduction in the insulin dosage often is necessary when a vigorous exercise session lasts ≥30 min. The specific adjustment that will be needed depends on the insulin dosage, the timing of exercise in relation to insulin "peak" action time, and the planned intensity and duration of an activity. For a moderate amount of exercise, a modest reduction (~20–30%) in the insulin component that is most active during the period of exercise may be sufficient to prevent hypoglycemia. However, for very prolonged, vigorous exercise such as distance running, cross-country skiing, cycling, or backpacking, a large decrease in the total daily insulin dosage (by as much as 50–80%) may be needed to prevent hypoglycemia. In this case, both short- or rapid- and longer-acting insulin may need to be decreased proportionally. Insulin reductions may also be necessary during the postexercise recovery period.

An elevation in the preexercise blood glucose level can be an indicator of an insulin-deficient state. Supplemental insulin may be necessary to correct a low insulin level and improve metabolic control before exercise is initiated.

If an exercise session is to be initiated within 30 min of an insulin injection, the injection should be administered in an area of the body that will not predominantly be used for the activity. Insulin absorption and peak action time can be accelerated if insulin is injected into an area of working muscle shortly before initiation of exercise. The abdomen is generally the site of choice.

CONCLUSION

Long recognized as a cornerstone of diabetes management, exercise is an all too often underutilized therapeutic modality. Although exercise carries potential risks for people with diabetes, with careful planning, it can provide numerous health benefits that far outweigh these risks. Using established, sound guidelines, physicians and diabetes educators can frame safe and effective exercise programs that will enhance the health and well-being of individuals with type 1 diabetes.

BIBLIOGRAPHY

American College of Sports Medicine: The recommended quantity and quality of exercise for developing and maintaining cardiorespiratory and muscular fitness and flexibility in healthy adults (Position Stand). *Med Sci Sports Exerc* 30:975–991, 1998

American Diabetes Association: *Handbook of Exercise in Diabetes.* Ruderman N, Devlin JT, Schneider SH, Kriska A, Eds. Alexandria, VA, American Diabetes Association, 2002

American Diabetes Association: Physical activity/exercise and diabetes (Position Statement). *Diabetes Care* 26 (Suppl. 1):S73–S77, 2003

Centers for Disease Control and Prevention and the American College of Sports Medicine: Physical activity and public health: a recommendation. *JAMA* 273:402–407, 1995

Colberg S: *The Diabetic Athlete.* Champaign, IL, Human Kinetics, 2001

Devlin JT: Exercise in the management of type 1 diabetes. *Pract Diabetol* 17:12–16, 1998

Lehmann R, Kaplan V, Bingisser R, Bloch KE, Spinas GA: Impact of physical activity on cardiovascular risk factors in IDDM. *Diabetes Care* 20:1603–1611, 1997

US Department of Health and Human Services: *Physical Activity and Health: A Report of the Surgeon General.* Centers for Disease Control and Prevention, National Center for Chronic Disease Prevention and Health Promotion, Washington, DC, US Govt. Printing Office, 1996

Wasserman DH, Zinman B: Exercise in individuals with IDDM (Technical Review). *Diabetes Care* 17:924–937, 1994

Young JC: Exercise prescription for individuals with metabolic disorders, practical considerations. *Sports Med* 19:43–45, 1995

Special Situations

Highlights
Special Situations

DIABETIC KETOACIDOSIS

■ Diabetic ketoacidosis (DKA) is a life-threatening but reversible complication characterized by severe disturbances in protein, fat, and carbohydrate metabolism.

■ DKA is always due to insulin deficiency, either absolute (e.g., a previously undiagnosed patient or omitted insulin) or relative (e.g., too little insulin injected or antagonism by stress [counterregulatory] hormones).

■ Any major stress may precipitate DKA in a patient with diabetes who lacks sufficient circulating insulin.

■ The clinical signs and symptoms of DKA are listed in Table 4.1. They usually include polyuria, polydipsia, hyperventilation, dehydration, the fruity odor of ketones, and disturbances in the conscious state from drowsiness to frank coma.

■ The initial goal of therapy should be to correct life-threatening abnormalities, i.e.,
- dehydration
- insulin deficiency
- potassium deficiency

■ Frequent reexamination of laboratory indices is imperative, at minimum, every hour during the first 4 h and at least every 4 h thereafter.

■ Routine bicarbonate administration is not recommended. Potassium administration is recommended for all patients. Some patients may require more aggressive therapy.

■ The cause of DKA must be aggressively pursued. Potential complications of therapy and how to avoid them are outlined.

■ DKA often can be prevented, given appropriate patient education and prompt physician attention.

HYPOGLYCEMIA

■ Hypoglycemia is a common side effect of insulin therapy. Mild hypoglycemic reactions usually consist of autonomic (neurogenic or adrenergic) symptoms, e.g., tremors, palpitations, sweating, and excessive hunger. Moderate and severe reactions include autonomic as well as neuroglycopenic symptoms, e.g., difficulty thinking, confusion, headache, slurred speech, dizziness, somnolence, seizures, or coma.

■ Mild hypoglycemic reactions may produce only minimal disruption of daily activities. Moderate and severe insulin reactions may severely harm health and morale and should be avoided.

■ Certain circumstances favor development of prolonged, incapacitating, and occasionally life-threatening hypoglycemia, i.e.,

- hypoglycemia unawareness
- delayed treatment
- failure to notice symptoms because patient is sleeping or attention is elsewhere
- intensive glycemic control
- long duration of diabetes
- certain medications or drugs

■ The factors precipitating an episode of hypoglycemia can often be identified, allowing prevention of future reactions in similar circumstances.

■ Self-monitoring of blood glucose (SMBG) should be used to full advantage for detection and treatment of hypoglycemia. Changes in insulin injection, eating, or exercise schedules and travel call for increased frequency of monitoring.

■ Guidelines for treatment of mild, moderate, and severe reactions should be clearly understood by patient, family, and school and business associates.

■ Hypoglycemia may occasionally lead to rebound hyperglycemia and should be recognized and appropriately treated if it occurs.

PREGNANCY

■ Women with type 1 diabetes who receive optimal care by an experienced diabetes management team can expect a pregnancy outcome similar to that of women who do not have diabetes.

■ Excellent glycemic control during pregnancy has been shown to bring unequivocally beneficial results to both mother and fetus.

■ Poor perinatal outcome is associated with poor glycemic control, ketonemia, and vasculopathy.

■ Patients should be as near to normoglycemia as possible at the time of conception and throughout the 1st trimester to decrease incidence of congenital malformations.

■ Frequent SMBG is mandatory during pregnancy.

■ Most women with type 1 diabetes may be managed as outpatients throughout gestation.

■ Tests to assess fetal growth and well-being should be conducted at appropriate times (Table 4.9). Timing of delivery, management during labor and delivery, and postpartum care are covered. Family planning and contraception must be reviewed with the patient during the postpartum period.

SURGERY

■ Given appropriate preparation and management, patients with type 1 diabetes are subject to little more than normal risk during surgery.

■ Whenever possible, the patient should be in the best possible general health and glycemic control before a surgical procedure.

■ The objectives of glycemic management before, during, and after an operation are to prevent hypoglycemia and excessive hyperglycemia and ketoacidosis.

■ Because hypoglycemia is particularly dangerous, plasma glucose is generally kept between ~100 and 150 mg/dl (5.6 and 8.3 mmol/l) during and after the operation.

■ Intravenous insulin delivery is preferred during surgery, although subcutaneous insulin may be used if the patient has stable glucose control, the procedure is relatively minor, and recovery is expected to be rapid.

■ In patients with DKA who need emergency surgery, efforts should be made to delay surgery until DKA is treated.

■ Guidelines are given for
• major elective surgery
• major emergency surgery
• surgery with local anesthesia

Special Situations

DIABETIC KETOACIDOSIS

Diabetic ketoacidosis (DKA) is a life-threatening but reversible complication characterized by severe disturbances in protein, fat, and carbohydrate metabolism that results from insulin deficiency. DKA is considered to be a medical emergency requiring treatment in a medical intensive care unit or equivalent setting.

In DKA, the arterial pH is <7.2, plasma bicarbonate is <15 mEq/l, blood glucose is generally >250 mg/dl (>13.9 mmol/l), and ketones are elevated. DKA is always due to absolute or relative insulin deficiency. The counterregulatory or stress hormones include glucagon, catecholamines, cortisol, and growth hormone and are markedly elevated in DKA. Acting in concert, they antagonize the biologic effects of insulin and augment the metabolic derangements characteristic of DKA by promoting

- hyperglycemia secondary to increased glucose production and decreased utilization
- osmotic diuresis and dehydration secondary to hyperglycemia
- hyperlipidemia secondary to increased lipolysis
- acidosis secondary to increased production and decreased utilization of acetoacetic acid and 3-β-hydroxybutyric acid derived from fatty acids
- an increased anion gap secondary to elevated ketoacids and lactate

PRESENTATION OF DKA

The clinical diagnosis of DKA is usually apparent in a patient known to have diabetes. However, DKA may not be readily considered in new-onset diabetes. A blood glucose concentration <250 mg/dl (<13.9 mmol/l) usually excludes DKA unless the patient has been partially treated with insulin and fluids before presentation and has severely restricted his or her calorie intake.

Clinical Signs and Symptoms

The clinical signs and symptoms of DKA include polyuria, polydipsia, hyperventilation, and dehydration (Table 4.1). The fruity odor of ketones will be apparent, and disturbances in consciousness may vary from drowsiness to frank coma. Abdominal pain in association with an elevated white blood cell count and serum amylase may occur but resolves with therapy. If severe abdominal pain persists, a

Table 4.1 Common Presenting Symptoms and Signs in DKA

Symptoms	Signs
Nausea and vomiting	Dehydration
Thirst and polyuria	Hyperpnea or Kussmaul breathing
Abdominal pain	Impaired consciousness and/or coma
Somnolence	Fruity odor

surgical consultation should be obtained, because an acute condition such as appendicitis, bowel perforation, pancreatitis, or infarction may coexist and may have been the DKA precipitant.

Precipitating Factors

Any major stress may precipitate DKA in a patient with diabetes. Infections such as pneumonia, meningitis, gastroenteritis, and influenza are some of the many heterogeneous causes, as are trauma or myocardial infarction. In most patients, it is possible to identify a specific precipitating cause. Among the most common are deliberate or inadvertent omission of insulin. The latter is particularly common following interruption of insulin pump delivery because of the limited available depot insulin when only rapid-acting insulin is being used. Another common cause of DKA is secondary to mismanagement of sick days, i.e., withholding insulin from a patient who is vomiting and unable to eat and mistakenly believes this situation may result in hypoglycemia (Table 4.2).

ACUTE PATIENT CARE

The initial goal of therapy should be to correct life-threatening abnormalities, i.e., dehydration, insulin deficiency, and potassium deficiency. Fully correcting

Table 4.2 Points to Consider in Treating DKA

- A precipitating cause can be identified in most patients.
- An ECG is indicated in all adult patients.
- Isotonic saline is initially preferred to rehydrate patients.
- Intravenous insulin is the preferred route of delivery.
- DKA patients are deplete in total-body potassium.
- Administration of glucose is necessary to clear ketosis.
- Bicarbonate is rarely needed.
- Cautious replacement of phosphate is sometimes used.
- Preventing DKA is a long-term goal of sound diabetes management.

all biochemical abnormalities will take several days after the patient is eating. During the first 12 h of therapy, the condition must be reevaluated frequently. Particular attention should be paid to the plasma potassium concentration. A flow sheet tabulating successive changes in the patient's condition must be maintained for all patients (Table 4.3). The degree of hyperglycemia, acidosis, dehydration, and conscious state is variable. If the patient's clinical condition deteriorates after initial therapy has begun, help from an appropriate specialist is needed.

Therapy, laboratory data, and clinical assessment should be evaluated at presentation and monitored at frequent intervals for the first 12–24 h. Patients are generally best followed in an intensive care setting. For a recommended treatment schedule, see Tables 4.4–4.6.

Rehydration Process

Dehydration is present in all patients with DKA. There are many routes of water and/or electrolyte loss, including *1*) polyuria, *2*) hyperventilation, and *3*) vomiting and diarrhea. The best index of the degree of dehydration is the magnitude of acute weight loss, which may be determined if the patient's baseline weight is known. Other clinical indices include orthostatic hypotension, dry mucous membranes, decreased tissue turgor, and thirst. A decrease in urine output is less reliable because of persistent osmotic diuresis with hyperglycemia. It is reasonable to assume an average weight loss of 5–10% of total body weight.

Table 4.3 Ketoacidosis Flow Sheet

	Monitoring Interval
Clinical	
Mental status	1 h
Vital signs (T, P, R, BP)	1 h
ECG	Initially and as indicated
Weight	Initially and daily
Therapy	
Fluid intake and output (ml/h)	4 h
Insulin (unit/h)	1 h
Potassium (mEq/h)	4 h
Glucose (g/h)	4 h
Bicarbonate and phosphate (mEq/h)	4 h
Laboratory	
Glucose (bedside)	1 h
Potassium, pH	2 h
Sodium, chloride, bicarbonate	4 h
Phosphate, magnesium	4 h
BUN or creatinine	4 h

Adequate rehydration is extremely important in initial therapy. Isotonic saline (0.9% normal saline [NS]) is usually the initial choice of rehydrating fluid (Table 4.4). For patients who are hypertensive, hypernatremic, or at risk for congestive heart failure, a solution containing 0.45% isotonic saline may be preferable. In young children (age <10 yr), calculate fluid replacement according to body surface area, not weight (e.g., a 30-kg child has ~1 m² body surface area).

Insulin Replacement

Because the cause of DKA in all patients includes absolute or relative insulin deficiency, insulin must be provided. Insulin is required for suppression of ketone body production and is thus necessary to correct acidosis. Insulin also inhibits glycogenolysis and gluconeogenesis, suppresses lipolysis, and facilitates the conservation of sodium and other electrolytes by the kidney.

Only short-acting (regular) insulin should be used initially. Replacing insulin intravenously is the most direct route and is preferred if methods are available to regulate the infusion rate. Replacement via the intramuscular route is an alternative, but only if unable to do IV insulin (Table 4.5). Intravenous therapy may be started with a bolus dose of insulin (0.1 unit/kg) while setting up the insulin infusion as outlined in Table 4.5. This titration method will adapt to any degree of insulin resistance and prevent severe hypoglycemia as insulin resistance wanes.

Insulin and glucose infusion must be continued until both hyperglycemia and acidosis are corrected. Not giving glucose will delay clearing acidosis. Therefore, when blood glucose levels approach <250 mg/dl (13.9 mmol/l), 5% glucose with half NS plus potassium should be the rehydrating fluid with variable dose insulin by piggyback to maintain glucose in the target range. Some clinicians, particularly those treating patients in the pediatric age range, recommend moderating the target to a 200-mg/dl (11.1-mmol/l) range for 12 h, fearing that more aggressive treatment increases the risk of cerebral edema.

Table 4.4 Fluid Replacement

Hour 1–2

Provide 15 ml/kg isotonic saline (0.9% normal saline [NS]) or 500 ml/m⁻²/h; if patient has heart disease, administer fluid cautiously, e.g., according to central venous pressure.

Hour 3–4

Reduce fluid rate to 7.5 ml/kg/h in adults or 250 ml/m⁻²/24 h in children.
Adjust fluid rate to meet clinical need. Consider rate of urine output in fluid replacement calculation.

When blood glucose reaches 250 mg/dl (13.9 mmol/l), change fluid to 5% dextrose in 0.45% NS at 150–250 ml/h.

Continue intravenous fluids, including insulin, until acidosis is corrected. Then change to short- or rapid-acting insulin subcutaneously every 4 h, giving first dose 2 h before discontinuing intravenous insulin.

Potassium Replacement

Patients with DKA are depleted in total body potassium despite a normal or even elevated serum potassium level. The reasons for this are complex and include the catabolic state, potassium wasting in urine secondary to polyuria, inability of the kidney to rapidly conserve potassium, and often, the effects of vomiting and/or diarrhea.

Correct potassium replacement requires both caution and timely action. The following procedure is recommended:

- Establish urine output to be certain the patient does not have renal failure.
- Send blood samples to the laboratory to measure serum potassium.
- Do an ECG to rapidly estimate whether hypokalemia or hyperkalemia is present (high peaked T-waves in hyperkalemia; low T-waves with U-waves in hypokalemia).
- Begin potassium replacement at the suggested rate (Table 4.6).
- When laboratory reports are available, alter rate if necessary with the goal of maintaining the plasma potassium level between 3.5 and 6.0 mEq/l at all times.

Table 4.5 Insulin Administration in DKA

Initially, use short-acting (regular) intravenous insulin only:

- Administer insulin as 50 units regular insulin in 500 ml 0.9% NS controlled with an infusion pump.
- Before connecting infusion tubing to patient, run 30 ml insulin solution through tubing to saturate tubing absorption sites.
- Piggyback insulin line into the IV fluid line.
- Deliver at a rate (unit/h) equal to
  (blood glucose [BG] mg/dl – 60) × 0.02 ([BG mmol/l – 3.3] × 0.02)
  where 0.02 is the sensitivity factor (SF)
- Monitor BG hourly and adjust rate per formula.
- If BG is not decreasing, increase SF by 0.01 hourly until BG <150 mg/dl (<8.3 mmol/l).
- Maintain SF constant while BG 100–150 mg/dl (5.5–8.3 mmol/l).
- If BG <100 mg/dl (<5.5 mmol/l), decrease SF by 0.01.
- If BG <80 mg/dl (<4.4 mmol/l), give IV D50 equal to (100 – BG mg/dl) × 0.4 ml
  [(5.5 – BG mmol/l) × 0.4 ml].
- Maintain BG in 100–150 mg/dl (5.5–8.3 mmol/l) until DKA resolved.

Intramuscular route recommended only if no method is available to regulate IV insulin infusion rate:

- First hour of therapy, inject 0.5 unit/kg.
- Each hour thereafter, inject 0.1 unit/kg until BG is reduced to 250 mg/dl (13.9 mmol/l).
- Every 2 h thereafter, inject 0.1 unit/kg as necessary to maintain BG concentration at 100–150 mg/dl (5.5–8.3 mmol/l).

Table 4.6 Potassium Replacement

- Initially, ECG may be used as a guide for plasma K+ concentration.
- Replacement of K+ is based on plasma K+ concentration. If K+ is
  <3 mEq/l, infuse ≥0.6 mEq/kg/h
  3–4 mEq/l, infuse 0.6 mEq/kg/h
  4–5 mEq/l, infuse 0.2–0.4 mEq/kg/h
  5–6 mEq/l, infuse 0.1–0.2 mEq/kg/h
  6 mEq/l, withhold until K+ is <6.0 mEq/l

- Add K+ to replacement fluid therapy.
- Recheck plasma K+ every 2 h if plasma concentration is <3.5 or >6 mEq/l.
- Administer K+ as K+Cl- or as potassium phosphate; do not exceed 90 mEq/24 h potassium phosphate because of danger of hypocalcemia.

Once insulin infusion is begun, potassium replacement should be attended to promptly. Insulin tends to lower serum potassium by enhancing its movement back into cells, and hypokalemia-induced cardiac arrhythmia may result. If there is anuria, potassium should be infused with special caution.

Bicarbonate and Phosphate Replacement

Although it seems reasonable to administer sodium bicarbonate to the patient with DKA to correct the metabolic acidosis with alkali, it is not clear whether the potential benefits outweigh potential risks. The potential harmful effects are accelerated reduction in plasma potassium concentration and exacerbated intracellular acidosis. For these reasons, routine bicarbonate administration is not recommended in most cases of DKA when pH is ≥7.1. With severe acidosis (i.e., pH <7.0), particularly when hypotension, shock, and arrhythmias are also present, bicarbonate should be given as an infusion of 1 mEq/kg over 2 h and then after checking plasma bicarbonate level. Repeat as needed until pH is >7.1.

Patients presenting in DKA are usually phosphate depleted. Furthermore, as with potassium, administering insulin enhances the movement of phosphate into cells, further reducing the plasma phosphate concentration.

There are pros and cons to administering phosphate, an ion important to many chemical reactions at the cellular level. One potential benefit is that hyperchloremia may be less likely to result when potassium is replaced as potassium phosphate instead of potassium chloride. However, administering too much phosphate can induce hypocalcemia. Therefore, calcium levels should be checked before phosphate is administered.

Although routine phosphate replacement has not been shown to be of benefit in the treatment of DKA, conservative potassium phosphate administration not to exceed 1.5 mEq/kg/24 h is usually recommended. The bulk of the potassium is administered as potassium chloride.

OTHER IMPORTANT CONSIDERATIONS

It is important to pursue other aspects of therapy while correcting the laboratory abnormalities. The cause of DKA must be pursued aggressively. The physician must be certain that there is no coexisting medical condition.

In several reported series of adult patients admitted to the hospital with DKA, infection was the most common precipitating factor. Therefore, depending on clinical signs and symptoms, a chest X ray plus culture of the urine, throat, sputum, and blood is warranted.

An ECG is mandatory to access potassium levels and also because myocardial infarction may precipitate DKA. The clinician should also carefully investigate all possible causes of abdominal pain.

For patients using an insulin pump, immediate, temporary discontinuation and subsequent changing of the infusion set apparatus after giving a manual correction bolus by syringe is critical. Malfunction of the infusion system is the most likely cause of DKA in those on pumps. It is also the most readily treatable cause of DKA.

In addition to determination of the cause of DKA, other supportive therapy must be considered. Ensuring an airway and inserting a nasogastric tube to drain gastric contents in comatose patients are strongly recommended to prevent aspiration pneumonia. Low-dose subcutaneous heparin (5,000 units every 12 h) is often recommended to prevent hypercoagulability, especially in elderly patients. However, data that demonstrate the benefit of heparin administration in DKA are lacking.

Be alert to complications of treatment. Potential complications directly attributable to the treatment of DKA must be anticipated.

- Generally, glucose will be normalized more quickly than acidosis. Premature discontinuation of insulin may result in persistence and worsening of ketoacidosis.
- Failure to give IV glucose at 5–6.25 g/h when blood glucose is <250 mg/dl (<13.9 mmol/l) will cause persistence of ketogenesis.
- Hypoglycemia can occur if the insulin infusion is not tapered as insulin resistance improves and glucose toxicity clears. If acidosis is still present, the insulin infusion must be continued.
- Cerebral edema and death may occur, particularly in children. Although the etiology of this complication has not been determined, some authorities believe that it is caused by correcting hyperglycemia too rapidly and the use of excessive amounts of hypotonic fluid.
- Nausea and vomiting from feeding the patient before gastric peristalsis has returned can result in aspiration pneumonia.

INTERMEDIATE PATIENT CARE

Intravenous fluid and insulin should be continued until vital signs are normal, acidosis has been corrected, nausea and vomiting have stopped, and the DKA precipitating factor has been controlled.

When subcutaneous insulin is begun, three points should be considered.

- Because subcutaneous insulin takes effect more slowly than intravenous insulin loses its effectiveness, the first subcutaneous insulin injection should be given 2 h before stopping intravenous insulin infusion.
- Extra short- or rapid-acting insulin, every 4–6 h for the first 24–72 h, should be used to meet the increased insulin demands of continuing stress surrounding DKA, to overcome "glucose toxicity," and to facilitate rapid

adjustment of the insulin dose to control blood glucose during this transition phase. The patient should be carefully observed to prevent recurrence of acidosis in the transition phase.

- The patient may remain mildly insulin resistant for several weeks, so the dose of subcutaneous insulin may exceed the patient's usual requirements.

PREVENTIVE CARE

Most often, DKA can be prevented, given appropriate patient education and prompt attention. All patients with diabetes should be performing self-monitoring of blood glucose (SMBG) regularly and urine or blood ketone testing when hyperglycemic (>250 mg/dl [>13.9 mmol/l]) or sick. Patients must be taught how to give appropriate corrective doses of insulin when they develop hyperglycemia. A proven method of doing this is to use their previously prescribed correction bolus formula and repeat the dose at 2-h intervals until hyperglycemia has cleared.

Patients on insulin pumps must know to change all their disposables, i.e., infusion set, syringe, and insulin, at the first evidence of hyperglycemia (>250 mg/dl [>13.9 mmol/l]) that is associated with ketones or does not respond to an initial correction bolus.

Patients must contact their physicians as soon as they become ill or have nausea and vomiting, fever, or persistent hyperglycemia and hyperketonuria. When contacted early, the physician is often able to treat DKA successfully by prescribing frequent injections of short- or rapid-acting insulin and by oral administration of fluids. It may also be possible to rehydrate and reinsulinize the patient in the doctor's office or emergency room, thereby preventing hospitalization.

However, when there is any doubt that the patient can be successfully treated in the home, office, or emergency room, hospitalization is indicated.

CONCLUSION

The pathophysiology of DKA can now be understood in the context of insulin deficiency and excessive counterregulatory hormones combining their effects to produce a severe state of life-threatening metabolic decompensation. Insulin, fluids, and electrolytes, given judiciously under appropriate guidelines in a hospital setting, form the cornerstone of treatment. A precipitating event such as infection, infarction, or accidental or deliberate omission of insulin must be identified and treated.

BIBLIOGRAPHY

American Diabetes Association: Hyperglycemic crises in patients with diabetes mellitus (Position Statement). *Diabetes Care* 26 (Suppl. 1):S109–S117, 2003

Barnes HV, Cohen RD, Kitabchi AE, Murphy MB: When is bicarbonate appropriate in treating metabolic acidosis including diabetic ketoacidosis? In *Debates in Medicine*. Gitniks G, Barnes HV, Duffy TP, et al., Eds. Chicago, Yearbook, 1990, p. 172

Bratton SL, Krane EJ: Diabetic ketoacidosis: pathophysiology, management, and complications. *Intensive Care Med* 7:199–211, 1992

DeFronzo RA, Matsuda M, Barrett EJ: Diabetic ketoacidosis: a combined metabolic-nephrologic approach to therapy. *Diabetes Reviews* 2:209–238, 1994

Genuth SM: Diabetic ketoacidosis and hyperglycemic hyperosmolar coma. *Curr Ther Endocrinol Metab* 6:438–447, 1997

Kaufman FR, Halvorson M: The treatment and prevention of diabetic keto-acidosis in children and adolescents with type 1 diabetes. *Pediatr Ann* 28:576–582, 1999

Kitabchi, AE, Umpierrez GE, Murphy MB, Barrett EJ, Kreisberg RA, Malone JI, Wall BM: Management of hyperglycemic crises in patients with diabetes mellitus (Technical Review). *Diabetes Care* 24:131–153, 2001

Kraut JA, Kurtz I: Use of base in the treatment of severe acidemic states. *Am J Kidney Dis* 38:703–727, 2001

Marshall SM, Walker M, Alberti KGMM: Diabetic ketoacidosis and hypergly-caemic non-ketotic coma. In *International Textbook of Diabetes Mellitus*. 2nd ed. Alberti KGMM, Zimmet P, DeFronzo RA, Eds. Chichester, UK, Wiley, 1997, p. 1215–1230

Rosenbloom AL: Intracerebral crises during treatment of diabetic ketoacidosis. *Diabetes Care* 13:22–33, 1990

Sperling MA: Diabetic ketoacidosis. *Pediatr Clin N Am* 31:591–610, 1984

Viallon A, Zeni F, Lafond P, Venet C, Tardy B, Page Y, Bertrand JC: Does bicarbonate therapy improve the management of severe diabetic ketoacido-sis? *Crit Care Med* 27:2690–2693, 1999

HYPOGLYCEMIA

The precise blood glucose level at which patients develop symptoms of hypoglycemia is difficult to define, but generally, symptoms do not occur until blood glucose is <50–60 mg/dl (<2.7–3.3 mmol/l). Clinical hypoglycemia is the occurrence of typical autonomic and/or neuroglycopenic symptoms with low blood glucose levels, and its symptoms are relieved by the administration of carbohydrate. Because of its sporadic and somewhat unpredictable nature and because of the need for rapid treatment, hypoglycemia is often self-diagnosed on the basis of predominantly autonomic symptoms and may be treated without documentation of the blood glucose level.

PATHOPHYSIOLOGY

Hypoglycemia occurs when there is an imbalance between the rate of glucose removal from the circulation (e.g., uptake into muscle) and the rate of glucose entry into the circulation (e.g., release of glucose from the liver or ingestion of nutrients). Clinically, this most often occurs when there is one of the following:

- a relative excess of insulin (which inhibits hepatic glucose production and stimulates glucose utilization by muscle and adipose tissue)
- a decrease or delay in food intake (which decreases the availability of dietary carbohydrate or gluconeogenic precursors)
- an increase in the level of exercise (which accelerates glucose utilization by muscle)

In healthy individuals, as the glucose level declines below normal (typically to 50–60 mg/dl [2.7–3.3 mmol/l]), a complex series of neuroendocrine events occur that raise the plasma glucose concentration back toward normal. Glucagon and epinephrine are thought to be the most important counterregulatory hormones in this process because of their prompt secretion and potent ability to stimulate the release of glucose from the liver. In addition, epinephrine can contribute to glucose recovery by reducing glucose uptake into insulin-sensitive tissues, and it is responsible for many of the autonomic warning symptoms of hypoglycemia (see below). The other major counterregulatory hormones—cortisol and growth hormone—generally are released more slowly than glucagon and epinephrine and appear to have a more permissive role in glucose recovery. Finally, endogenous insulin secretion is typically inhibited by hypoglycemia, also facilitating the rise in plasma glucose levels.

In contrast, the patient with type 1 diabetes has several abnormalities in this feedback system. First, the secretion of glucagon typically becomes deficient within the first 2–5 yr of diabetes. Second, with more prolonged duration of disease, epinephrine secretion may also be impaired as a result of the development of subclinical autonomic neuropathy. Finally, the rate of absorption of insulin from a subcutaneous depot is not regulated by normal homeostatic mechanisms, such as nutrient availability, and thus, it continues despite the presence of ongoing hypoglycemia. The combination of these and other factors makes the patient with type 1 diabetes particularly susceptible to the frequent development of hypoglycemia.

MILD, MODERATE, AND SEVERE HYPOGLYCEMIA

Symptoms of Mild Reactions

Mild low blood glucose reactions usually consist of tremors, palpitations, sweating, and excessive hunger. These symptoms are mostly mediated through the autonomic (adrenergic) nervous system. Cognitive deficits usually do not accompany mild reactions, and patients are capable of self-treatment. These mild symptoms respond within 10–15 min after oral ingestion of 10–15 g carbohydrate.

Symptoms of Moderate Reactions

Moderate low blood glucose reactions include neuroglycopenic as well as autonomic symptoms, e.g., headache, mood changes, irritability, decreased attentiveness, and drowsiness. Because of confusion, impaired judgment, and/or weakness, patients may require assistance in treating themselves. Moderate reactions produce longer lasting and somewhat more severe symptoms and often require a second dose of carbohydrate.

Symptoms of Severe Reactions

Severe low blood glucose reactions are characterized by unresponsiveness, unconsciousness, or convulsions, and typically require assistance from another individual for appropriate treatment. Approximately 5–10% of type 1 diabetes patients suffer one severe reaction each year that requires emergency measures such as parenteral glucagon or intravenous glucose.

Potential Effects of Hypoglycemia

Mild hypoglycemic reactions may produce only minimal disruption of daily activities. Hypoglycemia can cause hunger with consequent overeating, thus contributing to obesity or hyperglycemia.

In contrast, moderate and severe reactions may be seriously disabling in many ways, and blood glucose levels should be kept high enough to avoid them. Hypoglycemia that interferes with normal thinking makes taking a school examination an impossible task; riding a bicycle, driving a car, or operating dangerous machinery become potentially disastrous. Repeated or prolonged episodes may cause irreparable damage to the CNS, especially in very young children. Finally, such reactions should be avoided because of their deleterious effects on the morale of the patient and family members.

Some patients develop either a fear of hypoglycemia or an inappropriate lack of concern. Fear of hypoglycemia can lead to chronic overeating, undertreatment with insulin, or both. Maintaining blood glucose levels of 200–300 mg/dl (11.1–16.7 mmol/l) to avoid hypoglycemia increases the risk of metabolic complications, including DKA. In contrast, patients with a nonchalant attitude toward hypoglycemic reactions may maintain levels of blood glucose that are too low and will consequently be at greater risk for recurrent severe hypoglycemia. These patients can sometimes be identified by glycated hemoglobin (A1C) levels in the normal range.

Antecedents of Severe Hypoglycemia

Certain circumstances favor development of prolonged, incapacitating, and occasionally life-threatening hypoglycemia. Patients with hypoglycemia unawareness are always at increased risk for severe reactions. The counterregulatory hormone response to hypoglycemia and the autonomic symptoms tend to decrease after several years of diabetes so that neuroglycopenic symptoms become the first manifestation for many patients. β-Blockers and certain other medications may also diminish early warning signs.

Intensive insulin therapy also increases the risk of asymptomatic hypoglycemia. Although the increased frequency of low glucose levels can be attributed partly to the more stringent treatment goals associated with intensive regimens, it is now apparent that physiologic alterations occur in the patient's ability to secrete counterregulatory hormones, and thus, the ability to recognize and recover from hypoglycemia is clearly impaired. These observations emphasize the importance of SMBG in such patients to detect and prevent these asymptomatic reactions.

Several anecdotal and retrospective reports have suggested that the use of human insulin is associated with an increase in the frequency and severity of asymptomatic hypoglycemia. However, more carefully controlled, prospective studies generally have failed to support this observation. If a patient is switched from animal to human insulin, the diabetes management team should be aware that the more rapid onset of action and dissipation of human insulin may require readjustment of the insulin regimen or timing of meals to prevent hypoglycemia.

Delaying treatment is another common reason that mild hypoglycemia becomes more severe. Because early autonomic warning signs such as headache, hunger, mood or behavior changes, or weakness are not specific to hypoglycemia, they are frequently misinterpreted or overlooked. This is especially likely if the patient's attention is directed elsewhere, which may occur during strenuous activity. Hypoglycemia during sleep is particularly difficult to detect. The patient should be questioned for the presence of nightmares or nocturnal diaphoresis, and family members should be alert to unusual sounds or activity during the patient's sleep.

COMMON CAUSES OF HYPOGLYCEMIA

The factors precipitating an episode of hypoglycemia can often be identified by looking back over the events of several hours preceding the reactions (Table 4.7).

Inadvertent or deliberate errors in insulin dose are a frequent cause of hypoglycemia; other causes are changes in timing or schedule of insulin administration or meals. For example, sleeping later than usual for patients on fixed regimens is potentially dangerous because it disrupts the balance and timing between insulin and food. Changing insulin type from a short- to rapid-acting preparation or changing the insulin regimen can cause hypoglycemia because of more rapid absorption or other factors.

Vigorous unexpected exercise or activity is commonly associated with hypoglycemia. Aerobic exercise of prolonged duration or increased intensity can cause a reaction that occurs several hours after the activity ends or even the next day.

Table 4.7 Common Causes of Hypoglycemia

Insulin errors (inadvertent or deliberate)
- Reversal of morning and evening dosage
- Reversal of short- or rapid- and intermediate- or long-acting insulin
- Improper timing of insulin in relation to food
- Excessive insulin dosage

Intensive insulin therapy

Erratic or altered absorption of insulin
- More rapid absorption from exercising limbs
- Unpredictable absorption from hypertrophied injection sites

Changing insulin preparations or regimens

Nutrition
- Omitted or inadequate amounts of food
- Timing errors: late snacks or meals

Exercise
- Unplanned activity
- Prolonged duration or increased intensity of activity

Alcohol and drugs
- Impaired hepatic gluconeogenesis associated with alcohol intake
- Impaired mentation associated with alcohol, marijuana, or other illicit drugs

Alcohol, marijuana, or other drugs often mask a patient's awareness of hypoglycemia in its earliest stages. By inhibiting the liver's gluconeogenic capacity, alcohol also prevents the body's normal ability to provide glucose and restore low glucose levels toward normal. Some of the most severe hypoglycemic reactions occur during or after parties because the combination of physical activity and the use of alcohol or drugs can mask recognition of the problem and prevent the usual self-correction of hypoglycemia.

Anticipating and Preventing Hypoglycemia

Once a situation that leads to hypoglycemia is identified, adjustments or changing regimens (e.g., to an insulin pump) or raising the lower glycemic target can often be made to prevent future episodes.

Sleeping late. Although most patients on regimens of multiple daily injections can safely sleep an extra 30–60 min without particular adjustments, patients who oversleep more than 1 h may need to plan in advance to alter insulin or food intake. For example, if sleeping late is anticipated, a 10–15% reduction of intermediate- or long-acting insulin on the previous evening is an effective means of preventing hypoglycemia. However, it may also lead to excessive morning hyperglycemia. When the patient awakens, the entire day's schedule of insulin and meals is advanced in time. Even the next day's schedule may be affected. All patients should be cautioned against awakening and taking insulin without eating and then resuming sleep. However, awakening early, performing a blood glucose test, administering insulin, eating breakfast, and then going back to sleep is generally safe. Patients on insulin pumps can usually sleep late without a problem if their basal rate is set appropriately. Before doing so, it would be wise to check the basal rate periodically by skipping or delaying breakfast and observing the glucose changes every 2 h by SMBG.

Exercise. To compensate for increased caloric needs of exercise, increased absorption of insulin from exercising muscles, and increased insulin sensitivity induced by extra activity, several strategies to prevent hypoglycemia can be employed. Most important, the exercising patient should always have a source of short-acting carbohydrate immediately available.

If early signs of hypoglycemia develop during exercise, the exercise should be halted and an appropriate amount of carbohydrate eaten (Table 2.6). If similar exercise has previously resulted in hypoglycemia, patients can anticipate and prevent it by snacking before, during, or after exercise, depending on when the episode occurred. Decisions regarding the type and time of extra food can be made based on SMBG.

Alternatively, hypoglycemia can be prevented by anticipatory adjustments of insulin. For example, if a patient usually takes short- or rapid-acting insulin before breakfast but is planning to exercise after breakfast, the insulin dose can be reduced by 10–20%. This strategy may be preferable for patients who do not want to increase the size of a meal before exercise or who are overweight.

Role of SMBG

The availability of SMBG has made the detection and treatment of hypoglycemia practical, even in the subclinical range. Therefore, SMBG should be taught to all patients who do not already use it, and its frequency should be increased in patients with frequent hypoglycemia. Changes in insulin injection, eating or exercise schedules, travel, and other activities recognized as contributors to hypoglycemia call for increased frequency of monitoring. Patients should be instructed to treat asymptomatic hypoglycemia detected by SMBG.

TREATMENT

Mild Hypoglycemic Reactions

For mild reactions, ingesting 10–15 g carbohydrate works quickly to increase the blood glucose and stop classic symptoms. Several sources of short-acting carbohydrate exist (Table 2.6). Employing premeasured glucose products instead of juice or food is recommended because patients have a tendency to consume >15 g of juice or food when they have symptomatic hypoglycemia.

Hypoglycemic reactions that occur during the night should be treated initially with 10–15 g carbohydrate followed by a longer-acting mixture of carbohydrate and protein, e.g., 8 oz milk, or 4 oz milk and a few crackers. This is intended to prevent further hypoglycemia during the night. This strategy also should be employed if the next planned meal is >1–2 h away.

Commercially available glucose tablets have the added benefit of being premeasured to help prevent overtreatment. Glucose gels or small tubes of cake frosting are convenient for children or patients who are uncooperative when hypoglycemic. Chocolate and ice cream should be avoided for treating acute hypoglycemia because the fat content retards absorption of available sugar and could contribute to weight gain from ingestion of unnecessary calories.

Because there is always a risk that mild hypoglycemia will progress to a more severe reaction, all episodes must be treated promptly. Patients should be instructed never to continue driving when they begin to experience hypoglycemia. They should stop, treat the hypoglycemia, and wait 10–15 min to do a blood test to ensure full recovery before they resume driving. They should always have with them their meter and glucose products with which to treat hypoglycemia.

Moderate Hypoglycemia

Individuals with moderate reactions will often respond to the oral carbohydrates listed in Table 2.6 but may require more than one treatment and take longer to fully recover. These patients may be alert but will frequently be uncooperative or belligerent. Under such circumstances, if it becomes difficult to cajole the patient to take oral carbohydrate, administration of subcutaneous or intramuscular glucagon may be more appropriate.

Severe Hypoglycemia

Patients with impaired consciousness or an inability to swallow may aspirate and should rarely be treated with oral carbohydrate. These patients require either parenteral glucagon or intravenous glucose. If these are not available, glucose gels, applied between the patient's cheek and gum, may be of some help.

Generally, clinical improvement should occur within 10–15 min after glucagon injection and within 1–5 min of intravenous glucose administration. However, if hypoglycemia was prolonged or extremely severe, complete recovery of normal mental function may not occur for hours to days. Repeated boluses of intravenous glucose do not hasten recovery unless blood glucose measurements show persistent hypoglycemia. If the hypoglycemic event was associated with convulsions, the postictal period may be associated with severe headaches, lethargy, amnesia, or vomiting. Decreased muscle control may also be seen and requires medical evaluation if it persists.

Recurrent episodes of severe hypoglycemia can lead to permanent cognitive deficits. To prevent recurrence, patients should eat their planned meal or snack (~10% of daily calories) after initial treatment of moderate or severe reactions or when treating any nocturnal reaction.

Glucagon. The dose of glucagon needed to treat moderate or severe hypoglycemia for a child <5 yr old is 0.25–0.50 mg; for an older child (age 5–10 yr), 0.50–1 mg; and for those >10 yr old, 1 mg. Glucagon should be given intramuscularly or subcutaneously in the deltoid or anterior thigh region. Parents, roommates, and spouses should be taught how to mix, draw up, and administer glucagon so that they are properly prepared for emergency situations. Kits that include a syringe prefilled with diluting fluid are available.

Intravenous glucose. If medical staff and equipment are available, intravenous glucose should be given as a primary treatment in preference to glucagon. The usual dose is 10–25 g administered as 50% dextrose over 1–3 min. A useful formula for giving 50% dextrose in the hospital is

cc of D50 = (100 – blood glucose mg/dl) × 0.4 ([5.5 – glucose mmol/l] × 0.4)

The dose can be titrated according to the patient's response. After the bolus injection, intravenous glucose (5–10 g/h) should be continued until the patient has fully recovered and is able to eat.

HYPOGLYCEMIA UNAWARENESS

In the Diabetes Control and Complications Trial (DCCT), about one-third of all episodes of severe hypoglycemia seen in awake, intensively treated patients were not accompanied by sufficient signs or symptoms so that patients could effectively prevent neuroglycopenia. In the past, hypoglycemia without warning was viewed as a rare condition associated with advanced autonomic neuropathy. This concept is incorrect. Forms of hypoglycemia without warning can occur in recently diagnosed patients, particularly in patients with repeated episodes of recent hypoglycemia and low A1C levels. Repeated episodes of hypoglycemia cause two problems. First, they blunt hormonal defense mechanisms that prevent hypoglycemia. Second, they lower the level at which early hypoglycemic symptoms are perceived.

The key clinical issue is that patients need to be reminded that the absence of symptoms of hypoglycemia when glucose level is <55 mg/dl (<3.1 mmol/l) should prompt consultation with an experienced physician. Increased reliance on more frequent blood glucose monitoring, particularly before driving and after strenuous exercise, should be considered. Recent evidence suggests that hypoglycemia unawareness can be reversed by intensive education and self-management training and efforts that successfully avoid hypoglycemia. These efforts may include adapting slightly higher blood glucose targets before meals and during the night (e.g., lower target to >100 mg/dl [>5.5 mmol/l]) and self-management training to help detect and prevent subtle early signs of hypoglycemia.

HYPOGLYCEMIA WITH SUBSEQUENT HYPERGLYCEMIA

Hypoglycemia followed by "rebound" hyperglycemia, also called the Somogyi effect, may complicate diabetes management in some patients. The phenomenon originates during hypoglycemia, with the secretion of counterregulatory hormones (glucagon, epinephrine, growth hormone, and cortisol). This hormonal surge, together with decreasing insulin levels, leaves counterregulatory hormones relatively unopposed. Hepatic glucose production is stimulated, thereby raising blood glucose levels. These hormones may cause some insulin resistance for a 12- to 48-h period. Moreover, excessive carbohydrate intake may be a major contributor to rebound hyperglycemia.

The frequency of this phenomenon is debated, and studies suggest that it is much less common than previously reported. It may follow nocturnal hypoglycemia, but it also may occur after hypoglycemia at any time. The hypoglycemic event that precedes the rebound may not produce sufficient symptoms to make it recognizable.

If rebound hyperglycemia goes unrecognized and insulin dosage is increased, a cycle of overinsulinization may result, i.e., more hypoglycemia, more rebound hyperglycemia, more insulin, more hypoglycemia. As a general rule, when hyperglycemia does not respond as expected to treatment adjustments, undetected hypoglycemia and rebound hyperglycemia should be considered as a possible explanation. Rather than increasing insulin dosage day after day, the clinician who suspects rebound hyperglycemia should endeavor to detect (via SMBG) and avoid the initiating hypoglycemic event.

Nocturnal rebound hyperglycemia should be investigated by measuring blood glucose levels between 2:00 and 4:00 a.m. and again at 7:00 a.m. If blood glucose levels between 2:00 and 4:00 a.m. are <50–60 mg/dl (<2.8–3.3 mmol/l) and those at 7:00 a.m. are >180–200 mg/dl (>10.0–11.1 mmol/l), rebound hyperglycemia may have occurred. The increased blood glucose level may be exacerbated by the waning effect of the previous dose of intermediate-acting insulin or a prominent dawn phenomenon (see below). A decrease in presupper intermediate-acting insulin or its deferral to ~9:00 p.m. or a change to a basal analog (glargine) should prevent nocturnal hypoglycemia.

DAWN AND PREDAWN PHENOMENA

The amount of insulin required to normalize blood glucose during the night is less in the predawn period (1:00–3:00 a.m.) than at dawn (5:00–8:00 a.m.). The modest (20–40 mg/dl [1.1–2.2 mmol/l]) increase in plasma glucose commonly seen in patients with type 1 diabetes given enough insulin to avoid hypoglycemia in the predawn period is referred to as the dawn phenomenon. This increment can be greater if insulin levels decline between the predawn and dawn periods or if hypoglycemia occurs during the predawn period. The key clinical implication is that attempts to normalize prebreakfast glucose level (i.e., 70–115 mg/dl [3.9–6.4 mmol/l]) often result in predawn hypoglycemia.

Several strategies can be used to identify and prevent nocturnal hypoglycemia. These should include monitoring blood glucose at bedtime and at 2:00–3:00 a.m., especially when insulin doses are being adjusted to correct prebreakfast hyperglycemia or when blood glucose level is frequently in the normoglycemic range before breakfast. In the DCCT, >50% of all episodes of severe hypoglycemia occurred during the night or when patients were asleep, even with the use of long-acting insulin preparations given at night or insulin infusion pumps. As a consequence, the median blood glucose before breakfast was 140 mg/dl (7.8 mmol/l), and >75% of all prebreakfast values were over the upper target range of 120 mg/dl (6.7 mmol/l). Adding extra food at bedtime (particularly protein, which helps stimulate glucagon secretion) and giving insulin that does not "peak" at 1:00–3:00 a.m. should be considered. Increasing the bedtime snack is particularly important when nocturnal hypoglycemia is most likely (e.g., after sustained exercise during the day or when prebedtime glucose is <100 mg/dl (<5.6 mmol/l). Among patients taking twice-daily injections, giving the evening intermediate-acting insulin at bedtime or substituting it with long-acting insulin may be effective. Changing the regimen to an insulin pump can also help dramatically; the basal rate can be programmed to prevent nocturnal hypoglycemia as well as cover the dawn rise of glucose.

CONCLUSION

Severe hypoglycemia can be life threatening if not treated promptly. Even mild and moderate hypoglycemia can cause both short- and long-term problems. All patients should be taught to be aware of the signs of hypoglycemia and should be encouraged to use SMBG frequently to prevent and monitor episodes. All families should be taught how to use glucagon and when to call for medical assistance.

BIBLIOGRAPHY

American Diabetes Association: Hypoglycemia and employment/licensure (Position Statement). *Diabetes Care* 26 (Suppl. 1):S141, 2003

Amiel SA, Tamborlane WV, Sacca L, Sherwin RS: Hypoglycemia and glucose counterregulation in normal and insulin-dependent diabetic subjects. *Diabetes Metab Rev* 4:71–89, 1988

Bode BW, Steed RD, Davidson PC: Reduction in severe hypoglycemia with long-term continuous subcutaneous insulin infusion in type 1 diabetes. *Diabetes Care* 19:324–327, 1996

Bolli GB, Perriello G, Fanelli CG, De Feo P: Nocturnal blood glucose control in type 1 diabetes mellitus. *Diabetes Care* 16 (Suppl. 3):71–89, 1993

Clarke WL, Gonder-Frederick LA, Richards FE, Cryer PE: Multifactorial origin of hypoglycemic symptom unawareness in IDDM: association with defective glucose counterregulation and better glycemic control. *Diabetes* 40:680–685, 1991

Cryer PE: Hypoglycemia unawareness in IDDM. *Diabetes Care* 16 (Suppl. 3):40–47, 1993

Cryer PE, Fisher JN, Shamoon H: Hypoglycemia (Technical Review). *Diabetes Care* 17:734–755, 1994

Cryer PE, Gerich JE: Glucose counterregulation, hypoglycemia and intensive insulin therapy in diabetes mellitus. *N Engl J Med* 313:232–241, 1985

DCCT Research Group: Epidemiology of severe hypoglycemia in the Diabetes Control and Complications Trial. *Am J Med* 90:450–459, 1991

DCCT Research Group: Hypoglycemia in the Diabetes Control and Complications Trial. *Diabetes* 46:271–286, 1997

Fanelli CG, Epifano L, Rambotti AM, Pampanelli S, Di Vincenzo A, Modarelli F, Lepore M, Annibale B, Ciofetta M, Bottini P, Porcellati F, Scionti L, Santeusanio F, Brunetti P, Bolli GB: Meticulous prevention of hypoglycemia

normalizes the glycemic thresholds and magnitude of most of neuroendocrine responses to, symptoms of, and cognitive function during hypoglycemia in intensively treated patients with short-term IDDM. *Diabetes*
42:1683–1689, 1993

Havlin CE, Cryer PE: Nocturnal hypoglycemia does not commonly result in
major morning hyperglycemia in patients with diabetes mellitus. *Diabetes
Care* 2:141–147, 1987

Widom B, Simonson DC: Glycemic control and neuropsychologic function
during hypoglycemia in patients with insulin-dependent diabetes mellitus.
Ann Intern Med 112:904–912, 1990

PREGNANCY

Type 1 diabetes mellitus complicates ~0.1–0.2% of all pregnancies. During the past 25 yr, perinatal outcome has improved remarkably in this high-risk group. Except for deaths due to major fetal malformations, the perinatal mortality rate for women with diabetes who receive optimal care now approaches that of the general obstetric population.

Management of the patient with type 1 diabetes during pregnancy ideally involves an experienced medical management team, including the diabetologist or endocrinologist, obstetrician or maternal-fetal specialist (perinatologist), pediatrician or neonatologist, teaching nurse, dietitian, the patient, and her partner. Experience indicates that the outcome for both mother and baby is generally more favorable when an experienced team is responsible for management during pregnancy, delivery, and the perinatal period. When a team is not conveniently available, phone consultation with individual specialists is of paramount importance.

Pregnant women are usually highly motivated; therefore, this time is ideal for teaching self-care skills they can use for the rest of their lives.

RISK FACTORS

What factors help quantify maternal and fetal risk in pregnancies complicated by diabetes? Generally, risk factors fall into two categories: those relating to diabetes and its control and those relating to vascular complications. Thus, pregnancies complicated by type 1 diabetes can be divided into two groups: women with diabetes and women with diabetes and vascular complications.

Diabetes and Its Control

No longer does the onset and duration of diabetes influence the prognosis for good perinatal outcome. Instead, the degree of glycemic control at conception and the presence or absence of secondary nephropathy, vasculopathy, and hypertension greatly influence the prognosis for a favorable outcome for the mother and the fetus. The quality of maternal glucose control throughout pregnancy is also an important consideration. Poor blood glucose control, including ketoacidosis, is associated with intrauterine death.

Vasculopathy

The greater the degree of vasculopathy, the greater the likelihood of a poor outcome for mother and child. Nephropathy, particularly if associated with hypertension, appears to bring the greatest hazards, increasing the risk of preeclampsia, fetal growth retardation, and preterm delivery. Pregnancy can contribute to a worsening of retinal disease in women with background or proliferative retinopathy, especially in the presence of hypertension; women with active proliferative retinopathy are at greatest risk for progression, but visual loss can be minimized with laser therapy. Maternal deaths have been reported in patients with coronary artery disease. Other prognostically bad signs during pregnancy include ketoacidosis, pyelonephritis, preeclampsia, and poor clinic attendance or neglect.

MATERNAL METABOLISM DURING PREGNANCY

During gestation, maternal metabolism adapts to provide the fetus with an uninterrupted supply of fuel. During the 1st trimester of a normal pregnancy, accelerated utilization of glucose by the developing fetus generally produces a decrease in maternal glucose levels. In addition, pregnancy-associated nausea and vomiting can result in a decrease in food consumption. As a result, secondary hypoglycemia may occur unexpectantly and insulin requirements may decrease in the 1st trimester. Later in gestation, insulin resistance produced by the changing hormonal milieu may increase glucose levels, resulting in an increase in insulin requirement.

In nondiabetic pregnant women, glucose levels are often lower than those in the nonpregnant state. In pregnancy, human placental lactogen, prolactin, and progesterone alter maternal islet cell function, producing β-cell hyperplasia and contributing to maternal hyperinsulinemia. In addition, maternal cortisol is elevated during pregnancy, which potentiates glucose intolerance. Human placental lactogen (hPL), a growth hormone–like protein synthesized by the placental syncytiotrophoblast, produces insulin resistance and augments maternal lipolysis. As placental mass enlarges during pregnancy, hPL levels rise, allowing increased maternal utilization of fats for energy and sparing of glucose for fetal consumption. In late pregnancy, the progression of overnight maternal fasting ketosis is so accelerated that delaying breakfast may result in significant ketonuria.

In pregnancy complicated by diabetes, periods of maternal hyperglycemia produce fetal hyperinsulinemia. Larger amounts of maternal amino acids and other fuels also cross to the fetus. Elevated levels of maternal glucose and other nutrients stimulate the fetal pancreas, resulting in β-cell hyperplasia and hyperinsulinemia. This combination of fetal overnutrition and fetal hyperinsulinemia contributes to morbidity and mortality observed in the infant of the mother with diabetes.

PRECONCEPTION CARE AND COUNSELING

To prevent early pregnancy loss and very costly congenital malformations in infants of mothers with diabetes, optimal medical care and patient education and training must begin before conception. This is best accomplished through a multidisciplinary team comprised of a diabetologist, internist or family practice physician, obstetrician, diabetes educators, including a nurse and registered dietitian, and other specialists as necessary. Ultimately, the woman with diabetes must become the most active member of the team, calling on the other members for specific guidance and expertise to help her toward her goal of a healthy pregnancy and offspring.

Because treatment of the patient with type 1 diabetes must begin before gestation, any regular visit to the physician by a reproductive-age woman, from teenage to middle age, should be considered a preconception visit (Table 4.8). These contacts provide an important opportunity to discuss the patient's contraceptive needs and her thoughts and concerns about a future pregnancy and to establish a database that can be used in assessing perinatal risk. Adolescents in particular should be encouraged to discuss these issues routinely with members of the diabetes management team.

Table 4.8 Care Before Conception

- Discuss contraceptive program
- Establish database for perinatal risk
  Assess vascular status:
    Ophthalmologic examination
    ECG
    Exercise stress test if diabetes
      >20 yr duration
    Protein/microalbumin excretion
    Creatinine clearance
    Peripheral pulses
  Assess glycemic control via A1C testing
  Assess thyroid function: free T_4, TSH
    level, antimicrosomal antibodies

- Optimize glycemic control: A1C <6.5%;
  teach SMBG if needed
- Refer for assessment of nutritional adequacy; adjust if needed
- Determine immune status against rubella
- Evaluate psychosocial setting
  Caution patient against smoking or
    excessive alcohol
  Assess exercise program

Important periodic assessments include measurements of blood pressure, an ophthalmologic examination, an ECG, and a 24-h urine collection for creatinine clearance and protein/microalbumin excretion. Note that preexisting cardiovascular disease significantly increases morbidity and mortality to the mother. A1C testing should be performed routinely, and SMBG taught, if needed. The desired outcome of glycemic control in the preconception phase of care is to lower A1C (<6.5%) so as to achieve maximum fertility and optimal embryo and fetal development. To achieve these goals, the woman with diabetes must be empowered to take control of her own disease process. This requires effective patient education and integrated care by the diabetes management team in sharing knowledge of the rationale for tight metabolic control. Motivation for intensive self-management is dependent on the team's approach to imparting knowledge and skills to women with diabetes.

Immune status against rubella should also be checked before conception. Consultation with a nutritionist and a review of the patient's exercise program are important. The patient must understand that smoking and alcohol are strictly prohibited during pregnancy.

Because pregnancy complicated by type 1 diabetes may cause emotional and financial stress, it is essential to evaluate the psychosocial interactions of the patient and her partner, their support network, and their financial resources.

Women with type 1 diabetes who are contemplating pregnancy often have questions regarding its impact on their health and the possible consequences for the fetus. Some of the most commonly encountered questions, along with suggested answers, are presented below.

Q. How will pregnancy affect my life expectancy?

A. Pregnancy is not generally life threatening, but serious complications can occur if glycemic control is not maintained during pregnancy. There is no evidence that pregnancy shortens the lives of women with type 1 diabetes, except for some with established coronary artery disease. However, women with diabetes do face a higher risk for certain complications. If ketoacidosis occurs, there is the additional threat of fetal death. Preeclampsia and preterm delivery of the fetus by cesarean section are more common in women with diabetes.

Q. What effect will pregnancy have on diabetic nephropathy?

A. There is no evidence that pregnancy will permanently worsen diabetic nephropathy, although a temporary increase in proteinuria and decrease in creatinine clearance may occur. On the other hand, advanced nephropathy may jeopardize both mother and infant, increasing the risk for early preeclampsia requiring preterm delivery and/or a smaller-than-normal infant. Factors that point in this direction include

- proteinuria >2 g/24 h
- creatinine clearance <50 ml/min or serum creatinine >2 mg/dl
- hypertension: >130/80 mmHg despite treatment

Q. What effect will pregnancy have on diabetic retinopathy?

A. Except for women with active proliferative retinopathy, pregnancy is usually an ophthalmologically stable period. Women without diabetic retinopathy will not usually develop it during pregnancy. Very few women who have background retinopathy at the start of pregnancy experience a worsening of this condition and very rarely to a proliferative stage. Proliferative retinopathy treated by laser photocoagulation and stable before pregnancy will generally remain so. In contrast, many women with active proliferative retinopathy that has not been treated with photocoagulation experience a serious worsening of this complication during pregnancy.

Q. Will the baby develop diabetes mellitus?

A. The infant is slightly more likely to develop type 1 diabetes later in life because of maternal diabetes, but the risk is not very high, i.e., ~3%.

Q. Can I use birth control pills?

A. Young women without vascular complications may use a low-dose estrogen (≤35 µg)/progestin oral contraceptive. Those with hypertension or vasculopathy should use a progestin-only pill (or some other means of birth control).

Q. What effect will diabetes have on the baby?

A. The answer to this question appears to hinge largely on the mother's blood glucose control; generally, the better the diabetes control, the fewer the complications. In the first weeks of pregnancy, poor diabetes control appears to increase the occurrence of fetal malformations. Later, high blood glucose levels may bring about other serious consequences. Because glucose crosses from the mother to the fetus but insulin does not, high maternal glucose stimulates the fetus to overproduce insulin, which may

- cause excessive fetal growth
- prevent the baby's lungs (and other organs) from maturing at a normal pace

- give the baby serious hypoglycemia after birth, when it no longer receives glucose from the mother

In addition, high glucose levels are associated with sudden unexplained fetal death late in pregnancy.

CONGENITAL MALFORMATIONS: RISK AND DETECTION

The incidence of major congenital malformations is typically increased in the offspring of patients with type 1 diabetes over the 2–3% rate observed in the general population. However, the rate may vary considerably—from <5% in patients with excellent glycemic control before conception to as high as 20–25% among women with markedly elevated A1C in the 1st trimester.

Much evidence links such malformations with inadequate diabetes control during embryogenesis (gestational wk 3–7). The magnitude of risk for abnormalities of the brain, spine, and heart increases proportionally to the degree of elevation of A1C during this period. For this reason, patients should have as close to normal glycemic levels as possible at conception and throughout the 1st trimester. All women of childbearing age should be made aware of these risks, and if pregnancy is considered, they should be encouraged to use contraception until excellent glycemic control is achieved (see Philosophy and Goals, page 23). The risk of fetal anomalies should be reviewed at the first prenatal visit.

Fetal anomalies associated with diabetic embryopathy can be detected prenatally in most cases. The evaluation for a potential fetal malformation should include a maternal serum α-fetoprotein level at 16 wk, a detailed ultrasound examination of fetal anatomy at 16–18 wk, and an assessment of fetal cardiac structure by echocardiography at 20 wk (Table 4.9). All of these studies require interpretation by specialists experienced in prenatal diagnosis.

MATERNAL GLUCOSE CONTROL DURING PREGNANCY

Excellent control of maternal diabetes will reduce the risks of fetal demise, excessive fetal growth, and delayed pulmonary maturation. During a nondiabetic pregnancy, maternal plasma glucose rarely exceeds 100 mg/dl (5.6 mmol/l), ranging from fasting levels of 60 mg/dl (3.3 mmol/l) to postprandial levels <120 mg/dl (<6.7 mmol/l). These values should be therapeutic objectives for pregnancies complicated by type 1 diabetes (Table 4.10).

Table 4.9 Fetal Evaluation

Midpregnancy (16–20 wk): to detect fetal anomalies

- Maternal serum (α-fetoprotein)
- Ultrasonography
- Fetal echocardiography

Late pregnancy (28 wk to delivery): to assess fetal well-being

- Maternal assessment of fetal activity
- Nonstress test
- Contraction stress test
- Fetal biophysical profile
- Ultrasonography
- Lung profile by phosphatidylglycerol, lecithin-to-sphingomyelin ratio

Table 4.10 Target Blood Glucose Levels in Pregnancy

Time of Measurement	Blood Glucose (mg/dl [mmol/l])
Before breakfast	60–90 (3.3–5.0)
Before lunch, supper, and bedtime snack	60–90 (3.3–5.0)
1 h after meals	<120 (<6.7)
2:00–6:00 a.m.	60–90 (3.3–5.0)

A1C levels should be within the normal range for pregnancy (<20% of the nonpregnant range).

Maintaining maternal glucose levels in this range throughout gestation is difficult. During the 1st trimester, when morning sickness may be troublesome, the risk of hypoglycemia is increased; hypoglycemia is most likely during the night, when the mother is fasting but the fetus and placenta continue to consume glucose. In contrast, during the early 3rd trimester, when the diabetogenic stress of pregnancy is greatest, insulin needs may rise 50–100% over 4–6 wk, heightening the risk for ketoacidosis. The total insulin dose may double or even triple, compared with the prepregnancy dose.

Monitoring Control

SMBG. During pregnancy, women with type 1 diabetes must use SMBG to assess control. SMBG has been shown to decrease the need for hospitalization and reduce the cost of care. Patients should monitor in the fasting state, before each meal, and 1 h after meals. Testing at 2:00–3:00 a.m. is necessary for most patients, particularly for those who are likely to experience nocturnal hypoglycemia, those who have persistent fasting hyperglycemia, or those who are using continuous subcutaneous insulin infusion. The patient should be instructed to self-adjust insulin and maintain a careful record of the daily glucose and insulin values with comments about calorie intake and exercise.

Available data are too limited to permit specific recommendations regarding exercise programs in pregnant women with diabetes.

A1C testing. A1C testing should be obtained at the patient's first prenatal visit to assess previous glycemic control. This test should be repeated every 4–6 wk.

Ketone testing. Patients should be instructed to test for ketones any time glucose levels exceed 200 mg/dl (11.1 mmol/l).

Insulin Regimen During Pregnancy

An insulin regimen tailored to the patient's needs can be developed based on SMBG data, the meal plan, and the exercise regimen. Almost all women will require preprandial rapid- or short-acting insulin with a basal insulin. This may be any of the flexible regimens described in the Insulin Treatment section (page 51), except the basal insulin should not be glargine until it is proven safe in pregnancy. The greatest flexibility and control is provided by insulin pump therapy.

Some women may be controlled with a morning mixture of intermediate-acting and rapid- or short-acting insulins, rapid- or short-acting insulin before supper, and intermediate-acting insulin near bedtime. This regimen helps avoid glycemic irregularities overnight, decreasing the likelihood of nocturnal hypoglycemia and providing effective prophylactic treatment for the dawn phenomenon and/or the waning of the insulin effect in the early morning hours leading to prebreakfast hyperglycemia. However, postlunch glucose levels may be difficult to control without a prelunch injection of rapid- or short-acting insulin.

During pregnancy, most women prefer the flexibility of a four-injection regimen: a mixture of intermediate-acting and rapid- or short-acting insulins at breakfast, rapid- or short-acting insulin at lunch and supper, with an injection of intermediate- or long-acting insulin at bedtime.

In general, if glucose levels remain elevated pre- or postmeal, the corresponding insulin dose is increased by 10–20%. See *Medical Management of Pregnancy Complicated by Diabetes* (see Bibliography, page 157).

Insulin pump therapy. Pump therapy in pregnancy is best managed by a diabetes team with expertise in this form of therapy. Patients who have used insulin pump therapy before gestation should continue on this program. Patients who are not at goal either preconception or during pregnancy should be considered for pump therapy.

Pump therapy in pregnancy offers several advantages over multiple daily injections. Most important, quick titration of both basal insulin and bolus insulin to achieve the stringent goals of pregnancy without hypoglycemia is relatively easily accomplished. In times of morning sickness in the 1st trimester, the patient can rely on her basal infusion and take the bolus postmeal once the food is consumed. Boluses for snacks are also easily covered without the need of a separate injection. The increased need for insulin at dawn later in pregnancy is easily covered by increasing the basal rate during those hours. The pump also allows the nocturnal basal infusion to be decreased early in pregnancy if needed to reduce the risk of hypoglycemia.

Pump therapy is not without risks during pregnancy. Most important, should there be interruption of insulin delivery, rapid development of ketoacidosis due to the accelerated starvation characteristic of pregnancy may occur. All pregnant patients on pumps must be instructed at each visit how to troubleshoot hyperglycemia and change the infusion set and insulin reservoir if hyperglycemia (>200 mg/dl [11 mmol/l]) does not respond to a correction bolus. In addition, changing of the infusion site every two days is often needed in addition to rotation of the sites away from the abdominal area in the 3rd trimester. Skin irritation can be more common in pregnancy, and appropriate troubleshooting must be done.

NUTRITION NEEDS

The daily nutrition needs of pregnant women with type 1 diabetes should be based on a nutrition assessment by a dietitian. SMBG results, ketone tests, appetite, and weight gain can be a guide to developing and evaluating an individualized meal plan.

For most patients, 10% of the calories should be consumed at breakfast, 30% at lunch, and 30% at supper. The remaining 30% of calories can be distributed among several snacks, particularly a bedtime snack to decrease the risk of nocturnal hypoglycemia. Additional snacks may be added if the patient anticipates an increase in physical activity. Patients with persistently elevated midmorning glucose levels should reduce the calorie content of breakfast and redistribute the calories to lunch and supper. The presence of morning ketonuria with normal glucose levels indicates the need to increase the calorie content of the bedtime snack or to consider adding a snack around 3:00 a.m. However, there is no evidence that starvation ketosis has an effect on outcome. The calorie content of the meal plan may be reduced in women who are obese, who demonstrate early excessive weight gain, or who have a sedentary lifestyle. Guidelines for calorie needs for women who begin pregnancy at desirable weight can be obtained from appropriate references (see also Nutrition, page 85). Attention should be paid to providing sufficient intake of folate, calcium, other vitamins, and iron, although these vitamins and minerals are important for all pregnant women and not specific to women with diabetes.

OUTPATIENT CARE

Most women with type 1 diabetes may be managed as outpatients throughout gestation. Some may benefit from early hospitalization to evaluate cardiovascular and renal status and glucose control. Failure to maintain acceptable glucose levels, worsening hypertension, or infectious complications, such as a viral illness or pyelonephritis, may necessitate hospitalization. A urine culture should be ordered in the 1st trimester, because up to 25% of type 1 diabetic women can have asymptomatic urinary tract infections in the 1st trimester.

Clinic visits can be scheduled at 1- to 2-wk intervals for most women. At each visit, the patient's SMBG log should be reviewed, problems with hyperglycemia and/or hypoglycemia discussed, and the patient's weight gain and blood pressure checked. The patient should also be instructed to telephone the physician promptly if there are any episodes of hypoglycemia (<50 mg/dl [<2.8 mmol/l]) or hyperglycemia (>200 mg/dl [>11.1 mmol/l]) so that appropriate immediate remedial action may be taken.

Throughout gestation, the physician coordinating the patient's management must communicate regularly with other members of the medical management team. If background retinopathy has been detected, repeat ophthalmologic examinations should be obtained in the 2nd or 3rd trimester; proliferative retinopathy requires more intensive follow-up. If rapid normalization of blood glucose is needed, then monthly visits to the ophthalmologist are necessary to treat any development of neovascularization. Renal function studies, including creatinine clearance and protein excretion, should be repeated in each trimester if baseline values are abnormal.

Assessment of Fetal Condition

Significant advances have been made in the ability to assess fetal growth and well-being. The detection of fetal malformations between 16 and 20 wk is discussed above (see Congenital Malformations: Risk and Detection, page 150). In the 3rd trimester, attention should be directed toward the assessment of fetal well-being, growth, and pulmonary maturation (Table 4.9). Several approaches should be used to assess fetal condition to prevent sudden intrauterine death, a catastrophe most likely to occur during the final 4–6 wk of gestation.

Patient self-assessment. Maternal monitoring of fetal activity has proved to be a simple yet valuable screening approach in high-risk pregnancies. Daily assessment of fetal movement may be started at 28 wk gestation. The patient counts fetal activity for several 30- to 60-min periods throughout the day or records the time of day at which she has felt a total of 10 fetal movements. A significant decrease in fetal activity demands further evaluation.

Nonstress test. The nonstress test (NST) is an ideal screening technique that is easily performed in an outpatient setting and usually requires no more than 20 min. Fetal heart rate is recorded with an external heart rate monitor. A normal response is the presence of two or more accelerations of at least 15 beats and lasting at least 15 s during 20 min of observation. This "reactive" test is considered a reassuring finding. In a metabolically stable patient, a reactive NST will predict fetal survival for up to 1 wk.

The NST may be performed weekly after 28 wk gestation and then twice weekly at 32 wk of gestation. Because normal fetal activity and a reactive NST are rarely associated with an intrauterine fetal death, the primary value of surveillance is to allow the clinician to delay delivery safely while the fetus gains further maturity. However, because the screening tests have significant false-positive rates, an abnormal test, e.g., as a decrease in fetal activity, must be further evaluated.

Biophysical profile. Some clinicians have turned to the biophysical profile to assess fetal condition. The biophysical profile utilizes real-time ultrasound to observe fetal activity, fetal breathing movements, amniotic fluid volume, and fetal tone. Like the NST, the biophysical profile can usually be completed in 15 min and, if normal, indicates fetal well-being.

Assessment of Fetal Growth

Fetal growth should be assessed with serial ultrasound examinations every 4–6 wk. Delivery by cesarean section should be considered if the ultrasound suggests excessive fetal size In pregnancies complicated by diabetes, an infant >4,000 g increases the risk of shoulder dystocia.

The techniques utilized today for antepartum fetal surveillance permit most patients to remain outside the hospital even during the final 4–6 wk of gestation, as long as maternal control is acceptable and fetal evaluation is reassuring. Nevertheless, hospitalization may be necessary if the patient has nephropathy and/or hypertension, if she has not adhered to the regimen, or when fetal jeopardy is suspected.

TIMING OF DELIVERY

In the past, preterm delivery was often elected to avoid the risk of intrauterine fetal death. In many instances, such infants, although born alive, succumbed to respiratory distress syndrome (RDS). An increased incidence of RDS due to the combined effects of prematurity and diabetes, which may retard normal maturation of pulmonary surfactant production, was observed in infants of mothers with diabetes.

Today, delivery can be safely delayed until 38 wk in most pregnancies complicated by type 1 diabetes. Labor may then be induced after 38 wk without amniocentesis to confirm lung maturity, or the onset of spontaneous labor may be awaited. Patients must continue excellent glycemic control, and all parameters of antepartum fetal surveillance should remain normal.

In women who have vasculopathy, who have been in poor control, who have had a prior stillbirth, or who have not adhered to the program of care, early elective delivery to prevent a late fetal death may be planned provided that fetal pulmonary maturation has been confirmed by the analysis of amniotic fluid obtained by amniocentesis. RDS is highly unlikely when the amniotic fluid lecithin-to-sphingomyelin ratio is ≥2.0 and phosphatidylglycerol is present.

If the fetal lungs are immature, delivery may be postponed as long as the results of fetal assessment remain reassuring. It is essential that the obstetrician know the reliability of the analytical technique used for phospholipid analysis in the reporting laboratory, particularly in pregnancies complicated by diabetes mellitus.

Delivery despite fetal lung immaturity may be necessary when testing suggests fetal compromise or if the pregnant patient develops preeclampsia, rapidly worsening retinopathy, or renal failure.

LABOR AND DELIVERY

The timing and site of delivery must be discussed and coordinated with the neonatologists who are to be present. If delivery is anticipated and adequate maternal or neonatal care cannot be provided, the patient should be transferred to a hospital with an appropriately equipped nursery. Expert care is required to deal with the various complications that may arise in the infant of the mother with diabetes.

Intrapartum electronic monitoring of the fetal heart rate is mandatory. Labor should be allowed to progress as long as cervical dilation and descent follow the established curves for normal labor. Any evidence of an arrest pattern should alert the physician to the possibility of cephalopelvic disproportion and fetal macrosomia.

Maternal Glucose Levels During Delivery

Maintenance of normal maternal glucose levels (60–100 mg/dl [3.3–5.6 mmol/l]) during labor and delivery will reduce the risk of subsequent neonatal hypoglycemia. A glucose and insulin infusion can be used to maintain glucose levels in this range. During active labor in most patients, insulin requirements typically decrease substantially, with most patients requiring a reduction in their basal insulin. Glucose levels should be determined hourly with SMBG techniques at the bedside, because even small doses of insulin may produce hypoglycemia during active labor. Adjustments in the delivery of insulin and/or glucose should be made based on the glucose determinations. See *Medical Management of Pregnancy Complicated by Diabetes* (see Bibliography, page 157).

If labor is electively induced or a cesarean section is planned, the procedure should be scheduled for the early morning and the patient's usual morning rapid- or short-acting insulin dose withheld. If using an insulin pump, the basal insulin should be continued with suspension of the pump at the clamp of the cord to avoid maternal hypoglycemia. Epidural anesthesia is preferred in patients scheduled for cesarean section. After the operation has been completed, glucose levels should be monitored every 1–2 h, and an intravenous solution containing 5% dextrose should be continued. Because hPL and its contra-insulin actions fall rapidly after removal of the placenta, no insulin may be required for the remainder of the day if the previous injection of the long-acting insulin is still in effect.

POSTPARTUM CARE

In the immediate postpartum period, the patient's insulin requirements are usually lower than her prepregnancy needs. The antepartum objective of physiologic glycemic control is usually relaxed at this time and returned to prepregnancy levels (90–130 mg/dl [5.0–7.2 mmol/l]. If the patient uses an insulin pump, the basal rate should be reset at or below the prepregnancy rate. Breast-feeding is encouraged. The meal plan for the breast-feeding mother should be 30–37 kcal/kg desirable body weight.

If the patient delivered vaginally, and if glucose levels are ≥200 mg/dl (≥11.1 mmol/l), short-acting insulin should be administered as necessary as a correction bolus based on prepregnancy requirements. Once eating, the insulin regimen can be resumed but lowered to or below the prepregnancy insulin requirements. The doses should be adjusted based on SMBG.

In patients who have undergone a cesarean section, minimal insulin may be required for the first 2 postoperative days because calorie intake is limited. By day 2 or 3, the prepregnancy insulin schedule may be resumed and the dose adjusted using SMBG. Further adjustment of insulin needs in the postpartum period should always be individualized based on SMBG results.

FAMILY PLANNING AND CONTRACEPTION

Family planning and contraception must be reviewed with the patient during the postpartum period. Although oral contraceptives are the most effective method available, the increased risk of thromboembolic disease and vasculopathy require that combined estrogen/progestin oral contraceptive preparations be used with caution; only low-dose (≤35 µg) estrogen agents should be prescribed. Combination agents are contraindicated in women with hypertension or vasculopathy, who may be offered a progestin-only pill instead.

Motivated patients may do well with one of the barrier methods of contraception, such as the diaphragm, although their efficacy is significantly lower than that of oral contraceptives. Sterilization of the patient or her partner should be discussed with the patient when she has completed her family or if she has serious vasculopathy.

CONCLUSION

Advances in prenatal care and diagnosis, fetal surveillance, and perinatal care have markedly improved maternal and fetal well-being in pregnancy complicated by diabetes. Meticulous metabolic control before and during pregnancy holds the key to a successful outcome and to minimizing fetal malformations or perinatal complications. A team approach is more likely to achieve a desirable result.

BIBLIOGRAPHY

American Diabetes Association: Preconception care of women with diabetes (Position Statement). *Diabetes Care* 26 (Suppl. 1):S91–S93, 2003

American Diabetes Association: *Medical Management of Pregnancy Complicated by Diabetes.* 3rd ed. Jovanovic L, Ed. Alexandria, VA, American Diabetes Association, 2000

Jovanovic L, Fuhrmann K, Peterson CM: *Diabetes in Pregnancy: Teratology, Toxicology, and Treatment.* New York, Praeger, 1985

Jovanovic L, Peterson CM, Reed GF, Metzger BE, Mills JL, Knopp RH, Aarons JH: Maternal postprandial glucose levels and infant birth weight: the Diabetes in Early Pregnancy Study. The National Institute of Child Health and Human Development—Diabetes in Early Pregnancy Study. *Am J Obstet Gynecol* 164:103–111,1991

Kitzmiller JL, Buchanan TA, Kjos S, Combs CA, Ratner R: Preconception care of diabetes, congenital malformations, and spontaneous abortions (Technical Review). *Diabetes Care* 19:514–541, 1996

Kitzmiller JL, Gavin LA, Gin GD, Jovanovic-Peterson L, Main EK, Zigrang WD: Preconception care of diabetes: glycemic control prevents congenital anomalies. *JAMA* 265:731–736, 1991

Rizzo T, Metzger BE, Burns WJ, Burns K: Correlations between antepartum maternal metabolism and intelligence of offspring. *N Engl J Med* 325:911–916, 1991

Sommermann EM, Van Meter EK, Jovanovic L: Pregnancy and type 1 diabetes. In *Contemporary Endocrinology: Type 1 Diabetes: Etiology and Treatment.* Sperling MA, Ed. Totowa, NJ, Humana, 2003, p. 345–360

SURGERY

The physician caring for patients with type 1 diabetes mellitus must become familiar with perioperative management. With excellent glucose management, a person with diabetes can undergo surgery with little more than normal risk.

GENERAL PRINCIPLES

The objectives of glycemic management during surgery are to maintain normal glucose levels and normal metabolism. Insulin resistance and glucogenesis will increase during stress. For this reason, the customary basal insulin dosage is the minimum requirement during the perioperative period. Additional insulin also will be needed to prevent excessive hepatic glucose release and decreased peripheral utilization while maintaining normal glucose levels and normal fluid and electrolyte balance. Perioperative hyperglycemia will delay healing and increase the risk of ischemia. Plasma glucose levels between 100 and 150 mg/dl (5.5 and 8.3 mmol/l) during and after the operation are the target range. An operative/postoperative team guided by frequent point of care glucose monitoring, using a simple and safe algorithm for intravenous insulin administration, can maintain normal glucose levels and metabolism.

MAJOR SURGERY

Elective Surgery

The patient scheduled for elective surgery should be placed on intravenous insulin and glucose several hours preoperatively and maintained at 100–150 mg/dl (5.5 to 8.3 mmol/l). Evaluation of the metabolic state, lipid profile, renal function, and myocardial function must be completed before surgery. Once these procedures are done, surgery can be performed at any time of the day based on the urgency of the surgical condition.

Intravenous infusion of insulin rather than subcutaneous insulin administration is indicated during the perioperative period. Intravenous infusion allows careful control of the amount and speed of insulin delivery and circumvents problems with subcutaneous absorption in the event of shock. Suggested guidelines for management of patients with diabetes by use of intravenous insulin are found in Table 4.11.

Emergency Surgery

In the event of emergency surgery requiring general anesthesia, there is usually sufficient time to optimally evaluate and stabilize the patient. In the event of DKA in a patient who needs emergency surgery, e.g., trauma and ketoacidosis, the condition can be treated concurrently with surgery.

Table 4.11 Intravenous Insulin Regimen for Surgery

The simplicity of this regimen and the ease of adjustment of insulin or glucose infusion rates have made it the preferred mode of insulin delivery during surgery.

Preoperative Days

Attempt to obtain reasonable glycemic control, i.e., preprandial blood glucose (BG) concentrations 70–150 mg/dl (3.9–8.3 mmol/l).

Operative Day

Four to 8 h before surgery, keep patient NPO, omit usual subcutaneous insulin, and insert IV infusion line. Start infusion of 6.25 g/h glucose (125 ml/h D5 0.45% normal saline [NS] with 20 mEq KCl/l)

Administer insulin as follows:
- Deliver 50 units regular insulin in 500 ml NS controlled with an IV regulator pump.
- Piggyback insulin line into the D5 0.45% NS line.
- Deliver at a rate (unit/h) equal to (blood glucose [BG] mg/dl – 60) $\times$ 0.02 ([BG mmol/l – 3.3]) $\times$ 0.02), where 0.02 is the sensitivity factor (SF).
- Monitor BG hourly and adjust rate per formula.
- If BG is not decreasing or increases to >150 mg/dl (>8.3 mmol/l), increase SF by 0.01.
- If BG is <100 mg/dl (<5.5 mmol/l), decrease SF by 0.01.
- If BG is <80 mg/dl (<4.4 mmol/l), give IV D50W equal to (100 – BG mg/dl) $\times$ 0.4 ml or (5.5 – BG mmol/l) $\times$ 0.4 ml.
- Continue IV insulin as per formula with new SF.
- Repeat BG in 30 min.

After Surgery

- Continue IV insulin and glucose (D5 0.45% NS) infusion until 2 h after oral feeding is resumed. If patient is NPO for several days, infuse sufficient glucose (150 g/day in adults; 2–4 g/kg/day in children) to meet minimal catabolic needs. Adjust the insulin infusion as per above to maintain BG 100–150 mg/dl. (5.5–8.3 mmol/l).
- Transition to basal insulin glargine plus preprandial rapid-acting insulin when patient is able to eat.
- Insulin glargine should be given in a dose equal to the average rate per hour of IV insulin infusion over the past 2–6 h times 12, e.g., (120 – 60) $\times$ 0.03 $\times$ 12 = 22 units if the last multiplier was 0.03 and the average BG was 120 mg/dl.
- Rapid-acting insulin should be given after the patient has eaten and in proportion to amount eaten at 1 unit per 10 g carbohydrate. This will compensate for postoperative anorexia and nausea.
- Monitor BG before each meal, at bedtime, and 3:00 a.m.
- Correction doses of rapid-acting insulin should be given for any BG >150 mg/dl (>8.3 mmol/l), per the formula
  - Correction dose (U) = (BG mg/dl – 100)/correction factor (or [BG mmol/l – 5.5]/ correction factor)
  - Correction factor = 1700/(glargine units $\times$ 2 or average amount of insulin over the past 24 h). (Correction factor is usually 30 mg/dl [1.7 mmol/l].)
- For CSII patients: Resume basal rate and give boluses as per carbohydrate intake plus correction formula as above.

MINOR SURGERY

Patients undergoing elective surgery with local anesthesia (e.g., dental work) should eat only after surgery. The ideal management during these circumstances is to withhold food, withhold short-acting insulin, and continue basal insulin as insulin glargine or via insulin pump. If the person with diabetes is being managed in some other manner, they should be switched to a basal-bolus program before the elective procedure.

CONCLUSION

Medical management of the patient with diabetes requiring surgery must focus on provision of glucose and insulin in amounts to normalize blood glucose levels during and after surgery. Intravenous insulin and glucose at a rate adjusted for the individual's insulin requirement titrated from frequent blood glucose values will keep blood glucose levels between 100 and 150 mg/dl (5.5 and 8.3 mmol/l).

BIBLIOGRAPHY

Gill GV, Alberti KGMM: The care of the diabetic patient during surgery. In *International Textbook of Diabetes Mellitus.* 2nd ed. Alberti KGMM, Zimmet P, DeFronzo RA, Eds. Chichester, UK, Wiley, 1997, p. 1243–1254

Hirsch IB, McGill JB, Cryer PE, White PF: Perioperative management of surgical patients with diabetes mellitus. *Anesthesiology* 74:346–359, 1991

Husband DJ, Thai AC, Alberti KGMM: Management of diabetes during surgery with glucose-insulin-potassium infusion. *Diabet Med* 3:69–74, 1986

Levetan CS, Magee MF: Hospital management of diabetes. *Endocrinol Metab Clin North Am* 29: 745–770, 2000

Malmberg K, for the DIGAMI Study Group: Prospective randomized study of intensive insulin treatment on long term survival after acute myocardial infarction in patients with diabetes mellitus. *BMJ* 314:1512–1515, 1997

Pezzarossa A, Taddei F, Cimicchi MC, Rossini E, Contini S, Bonoro E, Gnudi A, Uggeri E: Perioperative management of diabetic subjects: subcutaneous versus intravenous insulin administration during glucose-potassium infusion. *Diabetes Care* 11:52–58, 1988

Richardson P, Steed RD, Davidson PC: Immediate correction of hypoglycemia without rebound using simple variable dosing of IV glucose (Abstract). *Diabetes* 48 (Suppl. 1):A363, 1999

Steed RD, Davidson PC, Bode BW, Sivitz WI: Computer controlled intravenous insulin infusion using intermittent bedside glucose monitoring: one year's experience (Abstract). *Diabetes* 35 (Suppl. 1):A32, 1986

Van den Berghe G, Wouters P, Weekers F, Verwaest C, Bruyninckx F, Schetz M, Vlasselaers D, Ferdinande P, Lauwers P, Bouillon R: Intensive insulin therapy in critically ill patients. *N Engl J Med* 345:1359–1367, 2001

Zerr KJ, Furnary AP, Grunkemeier GL, Bookin S, Kanhere V, Starr A: Glucose control lowers the risk of wound infection in diabetics after open heart operations. *Ann Thorac Surg* 63:356–361, 1997

Psychosocial Factors Affecting Adherence, Quality of Life, and Well-Being: Helping Patients Cope

Highlights
Psychosocial Factors Affecting Adherence, Quality of Life, and Well-Being: Helping Patients Cope

Diabetes is a demanding chronic disease. The diabetes management team must understand the patient's daily schedule, lifestyle, and developmental stage, as well as social and financial supports, when working to make diabetes management decisions and establish treatment goals. Maintaining quality of life is as important an outcome as good glycemic control.

PERIODS OF INCREASED EMOTIONAL DISTRESS

■ Emotional distress can be high at the time of diagnosis, when the honeymoon period is over, and at the onset of complications. Psychological equilibrium can generally be reestablished with early identification of distress; initiation of medical, psychological, and social supports; and monitoring of intervention effects. Initiation of multidisciplinary intervention can improve adaptation and adherence and prevent deterioration in metabolic control.

■ Monitoring of emotional status, quality of life, and well-being is an ongoing component of comprehensive diabetes care.

MAINTAINING ADHERENCE

■ Over time, regardless of age, motivation to maintain optimal diabetes control may wane. Maintenance strategies include planning a lifestyle-based diabetes regimen, improving patient/care provider communication, and employing research-tested educational and behavioral strategies (Table 5.2).

DIABETES COMPLICATIONS

■ Psychosocial factors should be suspected in the case of extreme poor control and/or recurrent diabetic ketoacidosis.

■ Repeat episodes of severe hypoglycemia can have serious psychosocial consequences, which call for medical, educational, behavioral, and family intervention.

■ When chronic complications begin, feelings of anger and guilt are common. Interventions that include psychological counseling and adaptive coping strategies can help resolve these emotional reactions. Family members should be included in the intervention whenever possible.

DEVELOPMENTAL CONSIDERATIONS IN CHILDREN

■ Although a diagnosis of diabetes during childhood can be a devastating experience for parents and children, families are usually resilient and adapt to the demands of the regimen within the first year.

■ Children's responsibilities for care should increase in tandem with cognitive and psychological maturity (Table 5.3). However, continued parental monitoring of care behavior is recommended throughout childhood and adolescence. Caution should be exercised in forcing too much self-care too soon or abandoning parental oversight during adolescence. Sharing diabetes care responsibilities produces the best glycemic outcomes and reduces individual burden.

DEVELOPMENTAL CONSIDERATIONS IN ADOLESCENTS

■ For adolescents, peer influences, together with family support and supervision, play an important role in adherence and glycemic control.

■ Many aspects of the treatment regimen are at odds with adolescents' normal drive for independence and peer acceptance. New technologies have enabled adolescents to maintain a flexible lifestyle but at the cost of increased monitoring and diabetes care tasks.

ADULTS

■ Misunderstandings about disability due to the disease can interfere with patients' attempting usual developmental tasks.

■ Adults with diabetes must deal with a disease and care regimen that complicates their interpersonal relationships and their attempts to establish a family and career, and presents a financial burden as well. Thorough and anticipatory education of patients, family members, and significant others can facilitate normalization of expectations.

THE ELDERLY

■ Older adults are an underserved population who can benefit from reeducation regarding newer technologies and care regimens.

■ The demands of the diabetes regimen may be especially burdensome for the elderly, who face other difficult life events such as retirement, loss of physical function, living on a fixed income, the death of a spouse and/or friends, and their own mortality.

■ The goal of diabetes care is to maximize physical and psychosocial functioning while respecting the patient's autonomy and independence as much as possible. Availability and maintenance of social support can be particularly difficult for the elderly, who often find themselves dependent on family and friends when physical capacities and financial resources diminish.

EMOTIONAL AND BEHAVIORAL DISORDERS AND DIABETES

■ Ongoing monitoring of the psychological status of patients will help with detection of diabetes-related distress and non–diabetes-related psychopathology. It is important to determine whether psychopathology is diabetes related or due to other causes.

■ Whenever possible, it is recommended that the care-provider team include a mental health professional familiar with diabetes and its care regimen.

■ Depression and anxiety disorders have been found to occur frequently in patients with diabetes. Some disorders, such as fear of hypoglycemia, needle phobia, and fear of complications and premature death, are specifically related to having diabetes.

■ Eating disorders should be suspected in individuals, especially young women with a history of unstable or poor metabolic control, recurrent ketoacidosis, or recurrent severe hypoglycemia, and in girls with growth retardation, pubertal delay, and/or amenorrhea.

STRESS AND DIABETES

■ Results of studies investigating the relationship between stress and blood glucose have been inconclusive. Stress responsibility is highly individualized.

■ It is important to establish a patient's stress reactivity to develop coping strategies to maintain good glycemic control up to, during, and after stressful events.

■ Stress can indirectly affect blood glucose control by undermining adherence to the diabetes treatment regimen.

Psychosocial Factors Affecting Adherence, Quality of Life, and Well-Being: Helping Patients Cope

Although type 1 diabetes taxes the patient's psychosocial well-being, the converse is also true: psychosocial factors can affect diabetes management. The unrelenting demands, inconveniences, frustrations of treatment, and possibilities of disability or death put tremendous emotional and financial strain on patients with diabetes and their significant others. Patients must struggle continuously to achieve a balance between the demands of their everyday lives and those of their diabetes regimen. To help patients cope successfully with diabetes in their everyday lives, the diabetes management team must consider the patient's daily schedule, lifestyle, and developmental stage, as well as social and financial supports, when making diabetes management decisions and establishing treatment goals. Maintaining quality of life is as important an outcome as good glycemic control.

PERIODS OF INCREASED EMOTIONAL DISTRESS

Psychological and emotional distress is high at the time of diagnosis, after the honeymoon period ends, and at the onset of complications (Table 5.1). At diagnosis, initial shock, denial, and anger often give way to mild depression and anxiety. Studies of newly diagnosed children and their families have found, however, that the initial reactions of both parents and children resolve rather quickly, and psychological equilibrium is reestablished within the first year. More extreme or long-lasting psychological reactions may indicate a need for referral to a mental health professional for evaluation and treatment.

Ongoing monitoring of the emotional status of the patient is part of comprehensive diabetes care. Initiation of an intervention as soon as emotional distress is identified may improve adaptation, prevent psychosocial maladjustment, improve compliance, and prevent deterioration in metabolic control. All members of the diabetes management team can be a great help during these periods by being accessible and sensitive to the patient's and family's need for information, support, and resources. When indicated, a referral to a mental health professional who specializes in working with patients with diabetes is suggested.

The following are suggestions for intervention aimed at facilitating adjustment and enhancing metabolic control.

- It is essential that the patient and his or her significant others are involved in the initial and ongoing discussions and education regarding diabetes care behaviors and regimens, lifestyle accommodations, sharing of diabetes care tasks, and the need to balance family needs with diabetes care tasks.

Table 5.1 Factors Causing Emotional Distress

- Uncertainty about the outcome of the immediate situation
- Feelings of intense guilt and/or anger about the occurrence of diabetes, poor glycemic control, and/or complications
- Feelings of incompetence and helplessness about the responsibility of managing the illness
- Fears about future complications and early death
- Loss of valued life goals and aspirations because of illness
- Anxiety about planning for an uncertain future
- Recognition of the necessity for a permanent change in living pattern as a result of diabetes

Adapted from Hamburg SA, Inoff GE: Coping with predictable crises of diabetes. *Diabetes Care* 6:409–416, 1983.

Both parents in the case of a child, the patient's spouse, the adult children in the case of an elderly patient, or any significant others should be included. This is important given the wealth of research showing significant associations between family and peer support and adherence, and problem solving and glycemic control. Research with families with children who have diabetes has shown that sharing diabetes care tasks and responsibilities reduces burden and can improve glycemic control.

- A comprehensive approach to diabetes education and management can be achieved if the roles of the diabetes management team are coordinated and regular communication takes place between care providers. Led by a physician or health professional who specializes in diabetes care, involvement of a nurse educator, a dietitian, a social worker, and/or a psychologist will ensure that the patient and family receive the educational, dietary, and psychosocial support they need.
- Self-management education with newly diagnosed children and their families in the months after diagnosis prevents deterioration in metabolic control during the first 2 years after diagnosis of type 1 diabetes. Close follow-up by the diabetes management team in the weeks after the initial education will increase, reinforce, and clarify diabetes knowledge. Furthermore, emphasis on developing self-management strategies during these weeks appears to enhance adaptation and metabolic control. Self-management education includes reinforcement of accurate glucose monitoring and recording and the use of these data to understand blood glucose fluctuations and make appropriate insulin and behavioral treatment changes. The goal is to help patients adopt a problem-solving approach to diabetes self-management. See also Patient Self-Management Education, page 32.
- Self-management education must be ongoing and accommodate the developmental lifestyle and agreed-on treatment goals of the patient and/or family members if the patient is a child, adolescent, or elderly person who requires assistance with care.

- Goals of treatment, diabetes care regimen tasks, and expectations for glycemic control should be negotiated with the patient and/or supervising adult so that unrealistic goals do not cause burnout and feelings of failure.

MAINTAINING ADHERENCE

Expectations that an individual and family will make multiple and significant behavior changes at one time may be unrealistic and unfeasible. Focus on "survival skills" at the time of diagnosis (self-monitoring of blood glucose [SMBG], insulin dosing, and monitoring of hypo- and hyperglycemia and ketones) and clear communication about the expectation of working toward intensive management of glucose control provide the foundation for success in diabetes self-management. A step-by-step approach to behavior change is often most successful, although highly motivated patients and parents will attempt to implement health provider recommendations when they are presented.

Failure to maintain self-care behaviors in diabetes management adherence and resultant poor metabolic control are frequently the result of the lack of attention to maintenance issues. Caution is needed to monitor burnout and feelings of being "controlled" by the disease. The strategies listed in Table 5.2 may help facilitate long-term adherence.

Individualized Treatment Regimens

Regardless of age, a patient's treatment regimen should be individually tailored. Patients have been shown to follow complex treatment regimens when the regimens meet the needs and requests of the patient and quality of life is maintained. Flexibility of lifestyle has become an important consideration in diabetes care, and advances in monitoring technology, insulins, and delivery systems have facilitated this aim. Holding a patient with diabetes to an inflexible diabetes care routine may increase the ease with which good glycemic control is achieved, but the negative impact on family and individual functioning should not be underestimated. The personality of the patient and his or her inherent organizational proclivities should help shape the diabetes care regimen that is adopted. Forcing a child or adult with attention-deficit hyperactivity disorder to keep detailed glucose records may be an exercise in frustration for all involved. Conversely, if such a patient prioritizes good glucose control, the diabetes care regimen may provide structure by which the individual organizes his or her daily routines. The adolescent, in particular, may be motivated to perform more frequent monitoring, take additional insulin injections, and adhere to a specific meal plan if it is perceived that he or she can participate in desired activities or be granted special requests. Conversely, many adolescents can attain improved metabolic control with better adherence to a simplified regimen than little or no adherence to a more complex or demanding regimen such as being placed on the insulin pump.

Negotiations regarding treatment regimens should be viewed by the care provider as an accommodation of the patient's treatment within lifestyle realities. Patients are people who happen to have diabetes. This is a departure from the philosophy of diabetes care in the past, which often presents difficulties for the care provider who wishes to provide a formula for success. Adoption of this point of view also helps providers avoid burnout and frustration with their patients.

Table 5.2 Strategies to Improve and Maintain Adherence

The Diabetes Care Milieu

- Provide a convenient office location and facilities that accommodate patients of all ages, with "child-friendly" areas set aside so that older patients are not disturbed or inconvenienced (if they so choose).
- Make appointment times as flexible as possible, utilizing after-school or -work hours whenever possible.
- Use appointment reminders that prompt patients to bring glucose records and meters.
- Maintain contact between appointments.

The Diabetes Management Team

- Increase communication between patient and team members by utilizing alternative methods of information transfer such as toll-free numbers, e-mail, or faxes.
- Elicit and discuss patient expectations for care behaviors, glycemic targets, and what to do when the regimen doesn't achieve the glycemic goals.
- Give specific instructions for self-care behaviors and problem-solving strategies whenever possible.
- Avoid jargon.
- Encourage questions and opinions from the patient. Let the patient/family know they are at the center of the diabetes management team and have equal voice in regimen decisions as long as sound medical practice is followed and good health is preserved.

The Regimen

- Involve the patient and family in treatment planning.
- Honor patient preferences and negotiate differences when planning the regimen and establishing treatment goals.
- Reduce the complexity and cost of the regimen when possible.
- Tailor the regimen to the patient's family lifestyle, culture, and finances.

Educational Strategies

- Update diabetes knowledge to keep pace with developing technology and changing patient needs, including developmental changes across the life span.
- Provide clearly written, easily understood instructions to reduce misunderstandings and forgetfulness. Make sure instructions are understood before the patient/family leaves the appointment.
- Use culturally relevant educational materials whenever possible.

Behavioral Strategies

- Encourage personal responsibility and problem-solving approaches.
- Negotiate realistic glucose and behavioral goals to be achieved between clinic visits (written contracts make these agreements more concrete).
- Attempt self-care behavior change in a step-wise fashion targeting one behavior until it is mastered. Relapse in behavior change is expected.
- Recognize and praise positive adherence behaviors and attainment of behavioral and glucose goals. Remind patients that setbacks are a part of diabetes care, not a failure.
- Continue to encourage family involvement and the use of community support mechanisms.
- Help patients identify and plan ahead for situations that might result in a lapse in adherence.
- Help patients develop coping strategies to prevent lapses in adherence to self-management behaviors.
- Help patients keep on track through follow-up phone calls, by responding to regularly mailed or faxed glucose records, and by using memory meters or glucose logs that allow the display of glucose trends and glucose averages over several weeks.

DIABETES COMPLICATIONS

Short-Term Complications

Recurrent diabetic ketoacidosis can be the consequence of underdosing or omission of insulin that occurs because of psychosocial problems, e.g., financial stress, parental neglect, lack of family involvement, chronic family conflict, weight concerns, or eating disorders. Psychosocial factors should always be suspected in the case of recurrent ketoacidosis, especially after it has been established that good glycemic control can be achieved under monitored conditions. A psychological/psychiatric evaluation should be considered for these patients.

Severe Hypoglycemia

Most patients with well-controlled type 1 diabetes experience several mild low blood glucose reactions each month. In general, these mild reactions, although distracting and uncomfortable, do not pose a serious problem for the patient. Severe hypoglycemia, however, defined as an episode in which patients are unable to treat themselves, lose consciousness, and/or have seizures, can be frightening and may have serious cognitive, neurological, and psychosocial consequences. The patient may develop fear of hypoglycemia and decide to maintain blood glucose values at unacceptably high levels. The family may also become overly fearful, watchful, or angry, blaming the patient for the disturbing episodes. Patients who experience severe hypoglycemia at work may jeopardize their job or chances for advancement.

Many patients with long-standing, well-controlled type 1 diabetes fail to recognize the early warning symptoms of hypoglycemia (hypoglycemia unawareness). These patients are at risk for repeated episodes of severe hypoglycemia and attendant medical and psychosocial consequences. Efforts should be made to prevent these episodes through reeducation and adjustments in the diabetes regimen (see Hypoglycemia, page 136).

The health care provider should discuss the patient's attitudes regarding hypoglycemia and help to establish safe blood glucose goals. Target blood glucose levels may need to be raised to restore hypoglycemic awareness and the patient's confidence in recognition of symptoms. A program called Blood Glucose Awareness Training (BGAT) successfully reduces the incidence of severe hypoglycemia. The family or significant others should be trained to recognize early or subtle hypoglycemic signs and provide adequate prevention and treatment measures, including the administration of glucagon. If the family is angry and blames the patient, the diabetes management team will need to help the family understand the difficulty many patients have in recognizing and avoiding hypoglycemia. The family should also understand that the patient frequently cannot control his or her behavior during a severe low blood glucose reaction.

Long-Term Complications

Although most patients are aware of the possibility of long-term complications of diabetes, the detection of the first evidence of retinopathy, nephropathy, or neuropathy can be a devastating event. When the onset of a severe complication occurs, the patient and family must cope with the grief associated with the potential or actual loss of body function. Once again, the patient and family may experience feelings of shock, denial, and anger. Feelings of anger at the health care provider for "letting this happen" or guilt ("I should have taken better care of myself") are common. These feelings can be eased by emphasizing the positive steps that can still be taken to forestall or prevent serious problems. When complications cause disability and restrictions in lifestyle, the treating physician or health care provider may need to refer the patient to a rehabilitation program that includes expert care or suggest counseling by an experienced mental health professional who is familiar with the disease and its treatment. Support groups or contact with people who have successfully adapted to complications can provide useful information and role models and help patients maintain a hopeful outlook.

Care providers and patients may be hesitant to broach the issue of sexual dysfunction—a common complication of diabetes in adults. It is critical to ask patients routinely about sexual function in a straightforward manner. Patients may be more likely to confide in the physician or another member of the diabetes management team if they know that sexual problems are common in diabetes and that a variety of treatment options are available. Along with issues of sexual functioning, issues of reproductive health should be addressed with teens, young adults, and adults of childbearing age. As diabetes care has enabled women with diabetes to have healthy babies, misinformation about the inevitability of poor pregnancy outcomes and the need to achieve excellent glycemic control before conception should be incorporated into routine diabetes care so that patients can make informed decisions regarding childbearing and fathering children.

DEVELOPMENTAL CONSIDERATIONS IN CHILDREN

Although a diagnosis of diabetes during childhood is a devastating experience for parents and children, families are usually resilient and adapt to the demands of the regimen within the first year. Some of those demands, viewed from a developmental perspective, are outlined in Table 5.3.

Generally, children's responsibilities for care should increase in tandem with cognitive and psychological development. Children who take responsibility for their diabetes care are generally more knowledgeable about their diabetes and are in better metabolic control. When treating a school-age child, the diabetes management team should be attuned to his or her cognitive maturity and abilities with regard to accurately interpreting results of SMBG, calculating carbohydrate intake, and preparing the correct amount of insulin. If cognitive abilities are questioned, referral for testing by a psychologist familiar with the treatment of diabetes should be considered.

Self-esteem is built through mastery of the developmental tasks of childhood and the positive regard of significant others. Children feel good about themselves when they succeed in tasks children their age are expected to master—school work, sports, social relationships, etc. Having diabetes presents children with opportunities to build self-esteem when they learn to perform diabetes-

Table 5.3 Developmental Issues and Tasks in Children with Type 1 Diabetes

Infant (0–1 yr)	Adopt a flexible care regimen that takes into account the infants variable appetite and activity levels.
	Differentiate hypoglycemic reactions from "normal" distress.
	Emphasize the necessity for frequent feeding, monitoring, and injections to control blood glucose and avoid hypoglycemia.
	Identify and train trustworthy babysitters to share diabetes care tasks and prevent burnout.
Toddler (1–3 yr)	Differentiate misbehavior ("terrible two's") from hypoglycemia.
	Expect dietary inconsistency as child begins to feed self.
	Give child choices in food, injection, and fingerstick sites (avoid mealtime battles).
	Encourage child to report "funny" feelings (hypoglycemia).
	Let child begin to "help" with diabetes tasks.
Preschool (3–5 yr)	Teach child to report hypoglycemia ("funny feelings") to adults in charge.
	Teach child what to eat when "low."
	Reassure child who may view fingersticks and injections as punishment and/or become overly fearful of procedures.
	Teach preschool teachers about diabetes, especially recognition and treatment of hypoglycemia.
	Encourage child to participate in simple diabetes care tasks such as "peeing on a stick" or placing a drop of blood on the meter strip.
	Involve child in menu planning.
School age (5–12 yr)	Teach all school personnel involved with child about diabetes.
	Optimize glycemic control to minimize school absences.
	Foster age-appropriate independence in diabetes-related and general social behavior.
	Parents and child should learn to adjust insulin and regimen to encourage participation in social and sports events.
	Encourage self-monitoring, recognizing hypoglycemia, and participating in meal planning; child should gradually learn to do own blood testing and injections, with all activities supervised.

Adapted from Schreiner B, Pontious S: Diabetes mellitus and the preschool child. In *Management of Diabetes Mellitus: Perspectives of Care Across the Life Span.* Haire-Joshu D, Ed. St. Louis, MO, Mosby, 1992, p. 362–398.

related tasks. These may be as simple as setting up supplies for blood glucose tests or as advanced as calculating the correct dose and giving their own injections or wearing and/or operating an insulin pump. This is especially true if parents, the diabetes management team, and others provide positive reinforcement for their achievements. Conversely, expectations of independent functioning in diabetes care tasks without the foundation of skill mastery, parental support and monitoring, and adequate time-management skills or structure can predispose the child to feelings of failure, low self-esteem, and feeling controlled by their illness. A child's comfort with self-care tasks should be monitored, because although a skill may be mastered, the child's desire to perform the task can change over time (e.g., during adolescence).

The Family

Diabetes affects every aspect of family life and affects all family members. Research has shown that shared responsibility within the family is associated with improved adherence and metabolic control. These results underscore the importance of educating family members regarding the treatment of diabetes and defining diabetes care tasks for each family member. Facilitating open discussion of the problems encountered in day-to-day diabetes management will help prevent blaming the child for poor diabetes control and enlist family support. Siblings, who commonly feel neglected or left out because of the extra attention given to the child with diabetes, may feel more involved if they are a part of the family's diabetes management effort, especially because they may be on the front lines with regard to recognition of hypoglycemia and its treatment. Fathers may be more likely to be involved if they, too, have clearly defined tasks. Full family involvement may help prevent overinvolvement of the mother and overly close dependence between the mother and the child with diabetes.

Diabetes, School, and Peers

School entry can be a difficult experience for parents and children. It is often more traumatic for the parent and child with diabetes, as they must now depend on teachers (who often are not knowledgeable about diabetes) to monitor the child's well-being and potentially handle situations that could be life threatening. The diabetes management team can help by providing diabetes literature and speakers for parents in their efforts to educate teachers, school nurses, and staff about diabetes. Many school nurses are now actively incorporated into the care regimens of their students with diabetes, and many take diabetes education and insulin pump classes to facilitate good glycemic control during school hours.

An important goal of diabetes management during childhood is to prevent the diabetes regimen from disrupting the child's school experience. Every effort should be made to ensure the child's safety at school. Recognition and treatment of hypoglycemia should be taught to school personnel. Protocols for specific diabetes-related issues, such as the timing of meals, exercise, and signs of moderate and severe hypoglycemia, should be generated by the treatment team and provided to the health liaison at the school. The diabetes management team should work with parents, teachers, and school nurses to minimize absences and missed class time and school activities. Children may quickly learn to use their diabetes to avoid difficult school situations. Educating school personnel about strategies that can correct low or high blood glucose levels will help prevent missed classroom time. Children who are frequently allowed to stay home for minor diabetes problems may fall behind in school and lose motivation to return to school. Social stigmatization can also occur because of being "sick" or "different." Every effort should be made to include children and adolescents with diabetes in all school-based activities, including field trips and sports.

During the elementary school years, peer relationships become increasingly important. This means that the diabetes management team must work with parents to ensure that children attend birthday parties and slumber parties, actively participate in school and recreation league sports, and participate in other normal childhood activities. This does not mean relaxing treatment goals. Use of long- and short-acting insulin and the insulin pump make adjusting to calorie, activity, and timing changes in the child's diabetes care routine feasible and straightforward. Adequate preparation and planning can allow the child to incorporate almost any usual childhood activity, including dosing of insulin for excessive calorie consumption or consuming extra calories for high levels of exercise. As stated in other sections of this chapter, quality of life is as important an outcome in diabetes care as good glycemic control.

DEVELOPMENTAL CONSIDERATIONS IN ADOLESCENTS

The adolescent years are known for difficulty with glycemic control, nonadherence to self-care regimens, and increased distress on the part of clinicians, parents, and the children themselves. Research has shown, however, that these difficulties can be lessened and that strategies can be developed to maintain glycemic control during this period of transition to early adulthood.

For the young child with diabetes, successful adherence to the treatment regimen depends largely on parental interest, management skills, and other resources. For adolescents, peer influences, together with family support and supervision, play an increasingly important role in adherence and glycemic control. Many aspects of the treatment regimen are at odds with adolescents' normal drive for independence and peer acceptance. Adolescents may neglect monitoring, dietary considerations, insulin administration, and even visits to the clinic to avoid drawing attention to their illness or disturbing their daily activities. These actions can have negative short- and long-term consequences, such as feeling sluggish and unfocused in the present, to chronically high blood glucose levels that can cause the onset of complications. The diabetes management team can use various strategies to help the adolescent patient and his or her family keep diabetes control within acceptable limits.

Understand the Scope of the Challenge

Almost all adolescents display characteristic behaviors and attitudes that reflect their drive for independence. Adolescents with diabetes are no exception. They undergo the same developmental process but with the added burden of diabetes. Do not assume that major difficulties are inevitable. There is no evidence that adolescents with diabetes suffer from serious psychological problems any more frequently than their nondiabetic peers. There is evidence that interventions can be suggested that are acceptable to the adolescent, parents, and health care providers that preserve glucose control and the adolescent's sense of autonomy. Use of the peer group and the diabetes management team to support and monitor the health status and behaviors of adolescents holds promise for affecting the decay in glycemic control often found during these years. Inclusion of the adolescent in devising a solution for nonadherence and/or poor control is highly recommended.

Many hormonal changes occur at puberty, some of which can adversely affect blood glucose levels. Puberty is associated with decreased sensitivity to insulin, which may result in increased insulin requirements. Poor control may be due to underinsulinization, lack of adherence, depression, or other psychopathologies or poor understanding of required health care behavior on the part of the adolescent. Do not assume nonadherence to care behaviors until good glycemic control has been achieved under supervised conditions utilizing the current insulin and diabetes care regimen. Blaming the adolescent for poor control can set the stage for further struggles with the adolescent and negatively affect communication, which is essential to problem solving. Empower the adolescent as an agent of his or her own good health outcomes.

Family and Patient Factors

Because family routines overlap with the various aspects of the diabetes treatment regimen (i.e., timing and content of meals, need for monitoring and exercise), family factors and adherence to treatment are strongly interrelated. Adherence to treatment is better among adolescents if their families are characterized by lower levels of general and diabetes-related conflict, greater cohesiveness (i.e., family members interact more and are supportive of one another), and clear assignments are made among family members for diabetes care tasks.

Effective clinical interventions with adolescents with diabetes and their families should target (for change) negative family interactions, especially those that focus on adherence with the care regimen. Whenever blood glucose values are outside of a target range, rather than blaming the adolescent, it is important for the family to problem-solve regarding the source of the poor glycemic control. Parents may need guidance in setting realistic expectations for their teen's self-management behaviors and blood glucose levels. Parents face a difficult balancing act wherein they must respect their teen's growing independence but remain responsible for their child's health and well-being. Negative family interactions may have the inadvertent effect of undermining the teen's attempts at independence in diabetes care. Education and problem-solving intervention efforts with adolescents should include parents, peers, and other acceptable support people, including the diabetes care team, at least as external monitors of glycemic status. Focus on the identification and development of coping strategies that decrease diabetes-related conflicts and tensions in the family and facilitate mastery of diabetes care skills is recommended.

Diabetes Management Team Factors

In addition to acquiring an understanding of normal adolescent development, members of the diabetes management team should enjoy working with adolescents and show a genuine interest in them as individuals. Patient valuation of their health care providers has been shown to be associated with better control. It is important for the diabetes care provider to directly interact with and involve the adolescent in their care, not just direct communication to parents.

Try to develop rapport. The diabetes management team should work toward rapport with the teen. Clinicians should avoid being placed in a parental role and make every effort to remain nonjudgmental and supportive in encouraging mastery and success in diabetes care behavior. Recommendations that are viewed by the adolescent as parental demands may be rejected. Clinicians are advised to adopt a child advocacy stance when interacting with adolescents, only assuming an authoritarian position when the child's health is at risk or risk-taking behavior is being demonstrated.

To avoid being viewed as parental figures, members of the diabetes management team should make it clear to both the parents and the adolescent that they have responsibilities to each other. The clinician may agree or disagree with either the parents or the adolescent about different aspects of diabetes care. An attempt should be made to convince the adolescent that the clinician-patient relationship is not one between clinician and child, but one between clinician and young adult.

Be willing to compromise. Each member of the diabetes management team must be willing to compromise on almost all aspects of diabetes care and must clearly demonstrate respect for the adolescent's views. If a clinician becomes frustrated and angry when the adolescent does not adhere to the regimen, it will be difficult to retain the ability to influence the patient's self-care. It is not necessary to agree with the adolescent's views, but the clinician should at least listen to the patient and make an effort to accommodate the patient's wishes whenever possible.

Be consistent. An important factor known to affect adherence across all age-groups is consistency in caregiving. The adolescent whose outpatient care is provided by any one of several different diabetes management team members with different management styles is not as likely to adhere to the regimen as the patient seeing a diabetes management team with a consistent and predictable management style. Often an adolescent will form a bond with one team member while professing to dislike another care provider. This may be face saving when the adolescent is nonadherent with care and gives health care providers the opportunity to play "good cop-bad cop." Ironically, this situation is often found in nonadherent adults as well.

Monitoring and Record Keeping

Adolescents and their parents are frequently at odds about monitoring and record keeping. At each clinic visit, the diabetes management team should negotiate with the adolescent on the type and frequency of SMBG as well as the kind of records to be maintained. New technologies, such as the combination insulin pen injector and meter, may be more acceptable to an adolescent and promote better adherence to blood testing. Adolescents (and others) who are seeking a way to avoid fingersticks and blood products in a public place (such as school) need to be made aware that alternative site testing (forearm) can be done but has its limitations.

When discussing the importance of monitoring to an adolescent, the diabetes management team should emphasize that it is done primarily for the patient's benefit and not to placate or please the parents or clinician. The adolescent should receive SMBG training (see Monitoring, page 77) independent of his or her parents and demonstrate independent mastery. Adolescents will be more likely to monitor and record their results if these results are used to make management decisions and are perceived as increasing flexibility and safety while maintaining metabolic control. It is important that if an adolescent becomes independent in SMBG, a mechanism must be set in place to communicate blood glucose results either to parents and/or health care providers independent of parental oversight.

Periodically, the adolescent patient may refuse to monitor at all. The heath care team should not give up. Instead, renegotiate. If the adolescent is willing to perform one test, another can be added at a future office visit. This step-by-step approach often yields good results among adults as well as adolescents. Stress to patients, however, that they need to resume monitoring if they become ill or are concerned about hypoglycemia.

Adolescents with diabetes commonly misrepresent glucose monitoring results. This is not surprising, given the many care demands, high parental and diabetes management team expectations, and the desire of the adolescent to be viewed as a "good patient." (Adults are less likely to "fudge" results, but may omit keeping records in the same spirit.) Misrepresentations can be of various types. One involves writing down results of tests never done. Another involves "editing" results so that undesirable values are "fixed," commonly by lowering high measurements. Yet another involves saving an old strip with a "good" reading and using this repeatedly to produce a desired pattern of glucose control. Misrepresentation should be suspected when the mean glucose values recorded are much lower than would be expected from a very high glycated hemoglobin (A1C) level or when safe round numbers appear to have been neatly recorded at the same time with the same pen.

After ruling out faulty measurement techniques and equipment and a form of hemoglobinopathy that would explain a higher-than-expected A1C level, misrepresentation of monitoring data for some secondary gain should be considered. When members of the diabetes management team suspect that home records misrepresent the facts, they should confront the adolescent with great care. Forcing a confession seldom serves a useful purpose. The diabetes management team should tell the patient that the blood glucose records are inconsistent with the A1C, and after ruling out other explanations for this discrepancy, urge the patient to be as accurate as possible in reporting blood glucose values. At the same time, the adolescent should be praised for testing and recording, even if blood glucose values are elevated. Also, they should be praised, not chastised, for leaving tests not done as blanks rather than filling them with fabricated values. No accusations should be made, and a problem-solving approach should be sought. This nonjudgmental approach may provide a good model for the parents, who should be encouraged not to punish the adolescent for having high but accurate glucose monitoring results. The diabetes management team should also remind parents that other adolescents with diabetes (and even adults) have problems adhering to the treatment regimen.

Parents often have great difficulty "letting go" of their role as primary manager of their child's diabetes. Parental worry for the child's well-being is to be expected, especially if parental responsibility for complications consequent to poor control have been warned against since diagnosis. Parents and teens may also be so used to interdependence in diabetes care that the child may view the parent as "not caring anymore" if they appear to withdraw from active participation in diabetes management. Unless the parent is assured that diabetes care tasks and reasonable glucose control are being maintained, they may be unable to let their adolescent proceed to independence in care. The need for communication, the method and frequency to be negotiated between parent and child, cannot be underestimated. Ironically, this developmental task is probably the most difficult of the adolescent years, and diabetes exacerbates the dilemma. Keeping the issue in a developmental framework can help patients, family members, and caregivers be more tolerant of the uncertainties produced by transition in care responsibilities.

ADULTS

Marriage, family, employment, and finances are four major aspects of adulthood. Adults with diabetes must deal with a disease that often complicates their interpersonal relationships and their attempts to establish a family and career and presents a financial burden as well. Adults are often not prepared to include the diabetes care team in the most intimate aspects of their lives, even though every aspect of their lives is affected by having diabetes.

Development of intimate relationships can be burdened by the self-care regimen of the individual with diabetes or by short- and long-term complications such as hypoglycemia or kidney failure. Men in particular may be hesitant to be in the patient role with their significant others or in their work environment. With the patient's agreement, the significant other can and should be incorporated into the diabetes care routine with proper education and knowledge of the treatment regimen. It is strongly advised that as a relationship becomes more important and central in a patient's life, the patient be encouraged to include the significant other in the diabetes care visits. It is especially important that the new person learn about the management of diabetes crises and methods of supporting adherence to the treatment regimen without demeaning the patient or treating him or her as disabled. Family planning counseling for couples planning a long-term commitment and the possibility of children will provide crucial information as the couple decides whether and/or when to have a child. Both partners should understand the risks of pregnancy for the woman with diabetes and the need for optimal metabolic control at the time of conception (see Pregnancy, page 146). Genetic counseling should be included with education to dispel misunderstandings about the genetic propensity to develop type 1 diabetes.

The diabetes management team should be able to help patients in many other ways during the adult years. They can offer education and counsel when misunderstandings and conflicts arise in a marriage because of diabetes; refer patients to community, state, and federal programs to help with financial problems; and educate and reassure children who worry about their parents' diabetes. Physicians can work with patients to match the regimen to the realities of their job and consult with employers if problems with diabetes management threaten a patient's job.

THE ELDERLY

Because of increased survival rates, there is a growing number of older adults with type 1 diabetes, in addition to the increasing number of older patients with type 2 diabetes who require insulin. The elderly are an underserved population and are often overlooked when new technologies and medicines are offered. The assumption is that more complex care is not feasible for this group of patients.

Many older people are active and functional and may wish to increase rather than decrease the intensity of their diabetes care. Retired people may have more time and resources to devote to diabetes self-care skills. Because of the availability of Medicare coverage, older people may have greater access to health services and be able to afford to participate more actively in their care. Ironically, the health care system may become a source of social support and routine for older patients.

The demands of the diabetes regimen may be especially burdensome for some elderly, especially those who face reduction in resources due to retirement, loss of physical function and mobility, the death of a spouse and/or friends, and their own mortality. It may be more difficult to keep physician appointments and purchase supplies because of transportation problems and financial limitations. Before assumptions are made about the needs or wishes of an elderly patient, a full current evaluation should be conducted that includes social factors such as interpersonal support, financial resources, and cognitive faculties. The diabetes management team should be aware that errors in insulin administration and blood testing may be due to failing eyesight or poor coordination, forgetfulness, or lack of understanding of new treatment modalities. It is essential for the diabetes management team to carefully assess each older patient to identify and address these potential barriers to sound diabetes care, and whenever possible to identify a support person who is willing to monitor the elder person's health status and provide concrete assistance.

Inevitably, there are changes in social support as one ages. Those who have helped in the past may no longer be able or available to do so. Social support is important to the health and well-being of older adults, but its role will vary by sex, race, marital status, and illness characteristics. It is important to determine the type of help needed to maintain respect for and autonomy of the older person. The goal is to provide support while safeguarding the patient's autonomy and independence as much as possible. Home-care agencies and special programs, such as Meals-on-Wheels, are often helpful.

As emphasized for other age-groups, the relationship between the diabetes management team and patient will influence patient adherence. Patients who are satisfied with their team are more likely to adhere to their diabetes care plan. However, older adults are less likely than other age-groups to express dissatisfaction directly to the provider. Therefore, it is even more essential to encourage open communication with this group by asking and responding to questions and by taking time to show concern and discuss problems.

EMOTIONAL AND BEHAVIORAL DISORDERS AND DIABETES

It is important that care providers recognize emotional and behavioral disorders in patients with diabetes and refer these patients for evaluation and counseling. Some caregivers mistakenly view psychiatric symptoms, especially those of depression and anxiety, as expected or even normal in people coping with an illness as serious and difficult to treat as diabetes. Unfortunately, when psychiatric symptoms are seen as the norm, therapeutic intervention may not be recommended, and the patient will continue to suffer psychological distress. This situation is especially disturbing in light of the high prevalence of depression and anxiety disorders in individuals with diabetes and the availability of effective treatment options.

Depression. Individuals with diabetes have higher rates of diagnoses of depression than the general US population and of other developed countries. It is not known whether depression predisposes to diabetes, glucose toxicity predisposes to depression, or some other central mechanism is operating that affects both conditions. Regardless, depression is still underdiagnosed, especially in teens and the elderly, and nonadherence due to depression is often mistaken for noncompliance with care recommendations. Ongoing monitoring of patients' mental status will help with prompt diagnosis and treatment. The use of multidisciplinary team care also has resulted in prompt diagnoses and initiation of care. When depression is suspected, referral to a mental health provider is recommended. Pharmacologic and behavioral treatments have both been shown to be effective in treating depression. As with all treatment of psychological and behavioral conditions, providers should be actively working with the diabetes management team to promote adherence and glycemic control. Incorporating the family and/or significant others into psychological care is also recommended.

Anxiety disorders. Anxiety disorders such as needle phobia and fear of hypoglycemia may be a consequence of treatment with insulin. Other disorders such as obsessive-compulsive disorder may be exacerbated by having diabetes. When symptoms are identified that suggest these disorders, referral to specialists who can initiate behavioral interventions while working with health care providers to maintain diabetes care behaviors is imperative. The goal is to prevent deterioration in metabolic control while reducing symptoms that limit the patient's ability to carry out diabetes care tasks. An anxiolytic medication in concert with behavioral intervention can also be utilized to diminish symptoms. Once again, it is important not to mistake anxiety for noncompliance, especially when the patient expresses distress in association with specific diabetes care tasks (such as injections).

Fear of hypoglycemia may result in patients wishing to raise their glucose levels to avoid the unpleasant feelings and loss of control associated with hypoglycemia. As mentioned above, BGAT has been shown to improve patients' recognition of their glycemic status and reduce the incidence of severe hypoglycemia. Other forms of behavior therapy, used while temporarily raising glycemic targets, can improve glycemic awareness in those who have lost feelings of hypoglycemia. Increased blood glucose monitoring and compensatory external cues can be enlisted to maintain glycemic status in those with hypoglycemia unawareness.

It is important to treat the disorders in addition to looking for compensatory management strategies (such as pump use and other methods of glucose monitoring besides fingersticks). Parents in particular often seek to avoid raising their child's anxiety level by "hurting" their child with insulin injections. This inadvertently promotes anxiety disorders and may solidify a child's fear. It is particularly important to include parents in treatment when children express anxiety over diabetes care behaviors.

Eating disorders. Eating disorders are common in (but not exclusive to) young women with type 1 diabetes and are associated with poor metabolic control, poor adherence to the diabetes regimen, and more severe complications. Eating disorders are often related to the regain of and increasing weight associated with successful treatment of diabetes with insulin. Diagnostic criteria for anorexia nervosa include weight loss and maintenance of body weight 15% below norm, impaired body image, intense fear of weight gain, and absence of menses. Diagnostic criteria for bulimia nervosa include recurrent episodes of binge eating, feelings of loss of control over eating during binges, frequent self-induced vomiting and/or laxative use, and overconcern with body image and weight.

Many young people with type 1 diabetes may have eating disturbances that compromise their diabetes control yet do not meet stringent diagnostic criteria. They may lose calories by intentional glycosuria rather than vomiting or laxative use. The seriousness of these subclinical cases should not be underestimated because they can result in short- and long-term metabolic complications. Eating disorders, clinical and subclinical, should be suspected in young women with persistently unstable or poor metabolic control, recurrent ketoacidosis resulting from insulin omission to induce glycosuria and weight loss, or recurrent severe hypoglycemia resulting from food restriction while continuing insulin and in girls with growth retardation and pubertal delay. These patients may require referral to an experienced mental health professional for psychological evaluation and treatment if an explanation for their problems is not found.

STRESS AND DIABETES

Although caregivers and patients have long observed a relationship between stress and blood glucose levels, the results of numerous studies attempting to define this relationship have resulted in contradictory results. Some studies have shown an association between stress and hyperglycemia, whereas others have not. In some studies, this relationship has been idiosyncratic, with patients varying dramatically in their glucose response to the same or different stressors. The only way to establish an individual's stress reactivity is to monitor blood glucose before, during, and after a stressful life event. Compensatory strategies should be developed according to the patient's individual response. Parents and teachers need to be made aware of a child's stress reactivity as it applies to schoolwork and sports activities to plan a strategy to achieve glycemic targets during stressful times in the child's everyday life.

Stress can also have indirect effects on diabetes. Patients under stress may be less able to follow their diabetes regimen, may give a low priority to their diabetes care, or may respond to the stress by overeating or increasing their use of alcohol or illicit drugs. Care providers should explore possible explanations for poor metabolic control. Some patients can learn to cope with stress management counseling or relaxation training.

BIBLIOGRAPHY

Anderson RJ, Grigsby AB, Freeland KE, De Groot M, McGill JB, Clouse RE, Lustman PJ: Anxiety and poor glycemic control: a meta-analytic review of the literature. *Int J Psychiatry Med* 32:235–247, 2002

Kovacs J, Brent D, Steinberg TF, Paulauskas S, Reid J: Children's self-report of psychologic adjustment and coping strategies during first year of insulin-dependent diabetes mellitus. *Diabetes Care* 9:472–479, 1986

La Greca AM, Follansbee D, Skyler JS: Developmental and behavioral aspects of diabetes management in youngsters. *Children's Health Care* 19:132–139, 1990

La Greca AM, Skyler JS: Psychosocial issues in IDDM: a multivariate framework. In *Stress Coping and Disease*. McCabe P, Schneiderman N, Field T, Skyler JS, Eds. Hillsdale, NJ, Erlbaum, 1991, p. 169–190

Lustman PJ, Anderson RJ, Freedland KE, de Groot M, Carney RM, Clouse RE: Depression and poor glycemic control: a meta-analytic review of the literature. *Diabetes Care* 23:934–942, 2000

Lustman PJ, Griffith LS, Couse RE, Cryer PE: Psychiatric illness in diabetes mellitus. *J Nerv Ment Dis* 174:736–742, 1986

Lustman PJ, Harper CTW: Nonpsychiatric physicians' identification and treatment of depression in patients with diabetes. *Comp Psychiatry* 28:22–27, 1987

Pontious S, Tesno B: Diabetes mellitus and the school-age child. In *Management of Diabetes Mellitus: Perspectives of Care Across the Life Span*. Haire-Joshu D, Ed. St. Louis, MO, Mosby, 1992, p. 399–440

Rodin M, Daneman D: Eating disorders and IDDM. *Diabetes Care* 15:1402–1412, 1992

Rodin G, Olmsted M, Rydall A, Maharaj S, Colton P, Jones J, Biancucci L, Daneman D: Eating disorders in young women with type 1 diabetes mellitus. *J Psychosom Res* 53:943–949, 2002

Surwit RW, Schneider MS, Feinglos MN: Stress and diabetes. *Diabetes Care* 15:141–142, 1992

Complications

Macrovascular Disease

Prevalence and Risk Factors
Assessment and Treatment
Symptoms and Signs of Atherosclerosis
Conclusion

Limited Joint Mobility

Detection and Evaluation
Conclusion

Growth

Mauriac Syndrome
Subtle Growth Abnormalities
Determining Growth Rate
Conclusion

Highlights
Complications

RETINOPATHY

■ Significant retinopathy in patients with type 1 diabetes rarely occurs before the 5th yr of the disease.

■ The clinician should evaluate the retinas of patients with diabetes with the direct ophthalmoscope annually even if no retinopathy is present and when indicated by symptoms or previous findings. Indications for more frequent ophthalmologic referral are described in Table 6.1.

■ The clinician should assure that patients receive their initial ophthalmologic examination within 5 yr of onset of type 1 diabetes (if >10 yr of age). Indications for more urgent ophthalmologic referral are described in Table 6.1.

■ High-risk characteristics of proliferative retinopathy greatly increase the risk of blindness and include

• new vessels on the optic disk (NVD) involving greater than ~25% of the optic disk area

• any NVD with preretinal or vitreous hemorrhage

• new vessels elsewhere covering an area ≥50% of the optic disk area (totaled for the entire retina) with preretinal or vitreous hemorrhage

■ When high-risk characteristics are present, photocoagulation therapy should generally be performed promptly. An eye with severe nonproliferative diabetic retinopathy, or worse, should be considered for photocoagulation.

■ Lesions typical of nonproliferative retinopathy, proliferative retinopathy, and macular edema are described in Clinical Findings in Diabetic Retinopathy (page 189).

■ Treatment for diabetic retinopathy can be highly effective in preserving or restoring vision. Treatment modalities include

• scatter (panretinal) photocoagulation

• focal/grid laser photocoagulation

• vitrectomy

■ Medical therapies are discussed in Treatment (page 194).

NEPHROPATHY

■ Epidemiologic studies have shown that up to 20–30% of patients affected with type 1 diabetes will eventually develop end-stage renal failure and require dialysis.

Complications

RETINOPATHY

Diabetic retinopathy is one of the four most common causes of blindness in the US and is a major cause of visual disability. Several surveys suggest that a person with diabetes has a 5–10% chance of becoming legally blind and that this risk is greater in people with type 1 versus type 2 diabetes.

Vision-threatening retinopathy virtually never appears in patients with type 1 diabetes in the first 3–5 yr of diabetes or before puberty. Retinopathy detected by fundus photography reaches a prevalence of 50% by the 10th yr. By the 15th yr, up to 28% of patients have proliferative retinopathy, in which new blood vessels develop from the retinal circulation, with a substantial risk of hemorrhage and traction detachment of the retina. After 20 yr duration of diabetes, nearly all patients have some form of retinopathy. Puberty, pregnancy, blood glucose control, hypertension, hypercholesterolemia, anemia, abdominal obesity, and cataract surgery may exert an accelerating influence on the development of retinopathy.

EYE EXAMINATION

Diabetic retinopathy appears primarily in the posterior retina and midperiphery. Many but not all lesions may occur within an area viewable by the nonophthalmologist with the monocular direct ophthalmoscope. Every physician should learn how to use this instrument. This examination is not an adequate substitute for an annual retinal examination by an ophthalmologist or optometrist who is knowledgeable and experienced in the management of diabetic retinopathy. It has been demonstrated that non–eye care professionals will miss a substantial amount of retinopathy, especially if pupils are not dilated. Although the finding of retinopathy by indirect ophthalmoscopy is well correlated with presence of disease and is important for prompt referral of the patient, lack of observed retinopathy does not obviate the need for comprehensive ophthalmologic evaluation in patients with diabetes.

Visualization of the retina is enhanced by dilating the pupils, which is easily accomplished in most patients with one drop each of 2.5% phenylephrine hydrochloride and 1% tropicamide. This procedure carries little risk in younger people, although there is an increasing risk of the ophthalmic emergency of angle closure glaucoma with advancing age and duration of diabetes. Blurred near vision and sensitivity to bright lights (requiring the use of dark glasses) are temporary inconveniences, lasting only a few hours, although patients should be warned not to drive until vision is restored.

CLINICAL FINDINGS IN DIABETIC RETINOPATHY

Mild to Moderate Nonproliferative Retinopathy

The earliest lesion visible through the ophthalmoscope is the microaneurysm, a pouch-like dilation of a terminal capillary. Ophthalmoscopically, microaneurysms look like tiny red dots. Dot hemorrhages may be indistinguishable

diagnose with the direct ophthalmoscope because this instrument does not allow the stereoscopic vision necessary to determine retinal thickening. However, the presence of hard lipid exudates—yellowish-white, often glistening, deposits of round or irregular shape lying within the retina, usually in the macular region—strongly suggests macular edema. This is particularly true if the exudates assume a ring-shape, or circinate, configuration. The features of clinically significant macular edema are

- retinal thickening at or within 500 μm of the macular center
- hard exudates at or within 500 μm of the macular center with adjacent retinal thickening
- retinal thickening >1 disk diameter in size any part of which is within 1 disk diameter of the macular center

Glaucoma

Sometimes, in advanced (usually proliferative) diabetic retinopathy, new vessels may also form on the surface of the iris and extend into the "angle" of the anterior chamber of the eye, where the cornea and iris come together (Figs. 6.5–6.8). Here, fibrous scar tissue extending from the new vessels may block the outflow of aqueous humor from the eye, causing a rise in intraocular pressure (neovascular glaucoma), severe pain, and loss of vision. Angle-closure glaucoma, a major complication, is a rare disorder in any age-group, especially before age 40 yr.

EVALUATION

The clinician should evaluate the retinas of patients with diabetes with the direct ophthalmoscope annually and when indicated by symptoms or previous findings. Patients with type 1 diabetes ≥10 yr of age should have an annual detailed ocular examination within 3–5 yr after the onset of diabetes. In general, this examination is not necessary before age 10 yr. However, some evidence suggests that the prepubertal duration of diabetes may be important in the development of microvascular complications, so clinical judgment should be used when applying this recommendation to individual patients. The examination should be done by an experienced ophthalmologist or optometrist and should include

- determination of visual acuity of each eye
- refraction, especially if visual acuity is impaired
- gross external examination of the eyes
- evaluation of ocular motility
- examination of the eyes by slit-lamp biomicroscopy
- examination of the retina with monocular direct and binocular indirect ophthalmoscopy after dilation of the pupils
- slit-lamp ophthalmoscopy to exclude macular edema
- in adult patients, measurement of intraocular pressures

In addition to undergoing the annual retinal examination by an ophthalmologist or optometrist who is knowledgeable and experienced in the management of diabetic retinopathy, patients with any level of macular edema, severe nonproliferative retinopathy, or any proliferative retinopathy require the prompt care of an

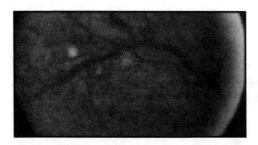

Figure 6.5 Severe nonproliferative diabetic retinopathy.
Note markedly dilated and
irregular veins. Beaded vein
extending from center to
11 o'clock looks like string of
sausages. There are multiple
blot hemorrhages and two
cottonwool spots just below
major vein in *center.* Fan-
shaped tuft of fine vessels
just above major vein (*right center*) may represent early neovascularization. Round, bright white spot above major vein (*left center*) is a photo-
graphic artifact.

Figure 6.6 Proliferative diabetic
retinopathy. Long, fine sprigs of
flat neovascularization elsewhere (i.e., not on optic disk;
also called NVE) arise in fan
shape from major vein in *center.*
Blot hemorrhages are in *upper
left.*

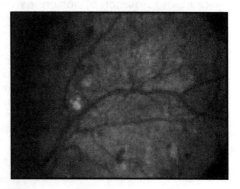

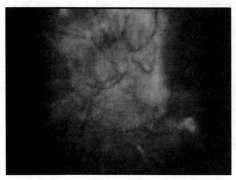

Figure 6.7 Proliferative
diabetic retinopathy. Extensive
fibrous proliferation extends
from optic disk, which is dimly
seen in center. Retinal vessels
are bent at right angles by
traction from proliferation.
Retina is partly detached, with
severe loss of vision.

ophthalmologist who is knowledgeable and experienced in the management of diabetic retinopathy. Some examinations should be carried out only for specific indications. These include retinal photography, which is used to document lesions, and
intravenous fluorescein angiography. During angiography, a fluorescent dye is
injected into a vein, and rapid-sequence photography of the retinal circulation is
carried out. Both eyes are typically evaluated at a single injection sequence.

Figure 6.8 Neovascularization of iris. This occurs in advanced, usually proliferative, diabetic retinopathy. Under normal conditions, blood vessels are usually not visible on surface of iris. Here, the extensive branching vessels of thick caliber, visible to left of pupil, are highly abnormal. They often grow

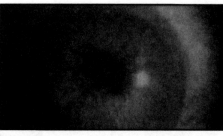

toward the iris periphery and into the filtration angle where they can occlude the angle where aqueous fluid outflow occurs. This produces extreme elevation of intraocular pressure, pain, and blindness. Pupil is irregular partly by contraction because of fibrous tissue and partly because of formation of posterior synechiae or adhesion between pupillary border of iris and underlying ocular lens.

Fluorescein angiography is useful clinically to plan photocoagulation treatment for macular edema. Although it is more sensitive than ophthalmoscopy or color photography for detecting very early lesions of retinopathy, the minute lesions detected are rarely critical for making decisions regarding treatment. Therefore, intravenous fluorescein angiography should not be used as a screening test in the annual ocular examination of patients with diabetes. Guidelines for care and referral are described in Table 6.1.

TREATMENT

Clinicians should always refer patients for treatment of retinopathy to an ophthalmologist, preferably one who is an expert in retinal disease (a retinal specialist). If laser treatment (described below) has been recommended, the clinician should check that the treatment has been implemented and that the patient maintains the recommended follow-up.

Photocoagulation

Scatter (panretinal) photocoagulation. The principle method used to treat diabetic retinopathy is by laser or light photocoagulation. For patients with proliferative retinopathy and HRC, scatter photocoagulation with the laser is standard therapy, based on DRS results and subsequent results from the Early Treatment Diabetic Retinopathy Study (ETDRS), another large-scale randomized controlled clinical trial.

In this procedure, a series of 1,200–1,600 (or sometimes more) laser burns, 500 µm in diameter and spaced one-half burn diameter apart, are placed throughout the midperipheral retina, avoiding the macular region. The DRS demonstrated that this procedure reduced the rate of progression to blindness by 50% in eyes with HRC over a 5-yr follow-up. The ETDRS study demonstrated that >95% of severe visual loss could be prevented if all patients receive scatter photocoagulation just as they exhibit HRC.

Many eyes with proliferative retinopathy but without HRC or with severe nonproliferative retinopathy also will require scatter photocoagulation. The fac-

Table 6.1 Guidelines for Care

Routine Care by Physician

- Examine retina with direct ophthalmoscope annually and when indicated by symptoms or previous findings

Referral to Eye Care Specialist

- Examine retinas through dilated pupils once a year (this need not be done before puberty unless the patient has eye symptoms or other complications of diabetes)

Referral to Ophthalmologist

- At the beginning of pregnancy or if planning pregnancy within 12 mo
- Moderate nonproliferative diabetic retinopathy, or worse
- Any level of macular edema (suggested by hard exudates within the macula)
- Immediate referral is mandatory (preferably to an ophthalmologist specializing in retinal disease) if any of the following are present:
  - NVD greater than ~25% of the optic disk area
  - any NVD with preretinal or vitreous hemorrhage
  - NVE ≥50% of the disk area with preretinal or vitreous hemorrhage
- Reduced vision from any cause
- Immediate referral is strongly urged when the following are present:
  - proliferative retinopathy without HRC
  - severe nonproliferative retinopathy, which includes
    - dilated irregular veins
    - multiple dot and blot hemorrhages
    - intraretinal microvascular abnormalities

tors determining whether such patients should receive treatment include type of diabetes, progression rate, contralateral eye status, systemic status, etc., and should be discussed with the patient by the retinal specialist.

Focal/grid laser photocoagulation. Diabetic macular edema is treated by focal/grid laser photocoagulation. With this technique, leaking microaneurysms and other vascular abnormalities in the macular region, determined by fluorescein angiography, are treated by direct application of small (50- to 100-μm) laser burns or laser burns placed in a grid-like pattern. The ETDRS showed that this treatment reduced the rate of visual loss from diabetic macular edema by 50% over a 3-yr follow-up.

Vitrectomy

Vitrectomy is a surgical procedure used primarily to *1*) remove vitreous humor filled with blood, *2*) cut fibrous traction bands, *3*) peel contractile fibrous membranes from the inner retinal surface, and *4*) repair some types of complex retinal detachments. Vitrectomy is particularly effective in certain cases of advanced proliferative diabetic retinopathy. Although it can often restore useful vision to eyes that would otherwise have severe visual impairment, vitrectomy is usually used only in more diseased eyes, as there are significant potential surgical complications.

Medical Therapy

It is important to maintain normal blood pressure levels and near-normal blood glucose levels in patients with retinopathy because diabetic retinopathy progresses more rapidly in patients with uncontrolled hypertension and hyperglycemia than in those whose blood pressure and blood glucose are normal. Control of systemic lipid levels is also important as dyslipidemia is associated with increased risk of hard exudates in the macula.

Therapies Under Evaluation

Other medical treatments for diabetic retinopathy have been evaluated.

- Aspirin (650 mg/day) was tested in the ETDRS because it inhibits platelet aggregation. Platelet microthrombi have been proposed as a factor in the cause of diabetic retinopathy. Aspirin was shown to be of no benefit or risk for retinopathy in this study.
- There is some evidence from animal experiments that two classes of drugs may be useful in preventing or reducing the progression of diabetic retinopathy: aldose reductase inhibitors and inhibitors of protein kinase C (β isoform). Although aldose reductase inhibitors have not yet shown good efficacy in clinical trials of retinopathy, recent clinical trials of protein kinase C inhibitors suggest they may help reduce macular edema progression and preserve vision. Definitive trials on the efficacy of protein kinase C inhibitors are underway.

CONCLUSION

Diabetic retinopathy is a common complication of long-term diabetes mellitus that ranks as a leading cause of blindness and visual disability. Appropriate care includes optimization of blood glucose, blood pressure, and serum lipid levels and routine, life-long ophthalmic examinations. Although treatment strategies cannot totally prevent or cure this complication, there is clear evidence that they can substantially retard its progression if used appropriately and provided promptly when indicated. Accordingly, careful evaluation of glycemic control and the ocular fundus of patients with diabetes by the primary care physician, together with annual or more frequent retinal examination by an ophthalmologist or optometrist who is knowledgeable and experienced in the management of diabetic retinopathy, is a standard of care for all patients with diabetes mellitus.

BIBLIOGRAPHY

Aiello LM: Perspectives on diabetic retinopathy. *Am J Ophthalmol* 136:122–135, 2003

Aiello LP, Cahill MT, Wong JS: Systemic considerations in the management of diabetic retinopathy. *Am J Ophthalmol* 132:760–766, 2001

American Diabetes Association: Diabetic retinopathy (Position Statement). *Diabetes Care* 26 (Suppl. 1):S99–S102, 2003

Cavallerano JD: A review of non-retinal ocular complications of diabetes mellitus. *J Am Optom Assoc* 61:533–543, 1990

DCCT Research Group: The effect of intensive treatment of diabetes on the development and progression of long-term complications in insulin-dependent diabetes mellitus. *N Engl J Med* 329:977–986, 1993

DCCT Research Group: The relationship of glycemic exposure (HbA1c) to the risk of development and progression of retinopathy in the Diabetes Control and Complications Trial. *Diabetes* 44:968–983, 1995

Diabetes Control and Complications Trial/Epidemiology of Diabetes Interventions and Complications Research Group: Retinopathy and nephropathy in patients with type 1 diabetes four years after a trial of intensive therapy. *N Engl J Med* 342:381–389, 2000

Diabetes Control and Complications Trial/Epidemiology of Diabetes Interventions and Complications Research Group: Retinopathy and nephropathy in patients with type 1 diabetes four years after a trial of intensive therapy. *Am J Ophthalmol* 129:704–705, 2000

Early Treatment Diabetic Retinopathy Study Research Group: Early photocoagulation for diabetic retinopathy: report number 9. *Ophthalmology* 98 (5 Suppl):766–785, 1991

Early Treatment Diabetic Retinopathy Study Research Group: Photocoagulation for diabetic macular edema: report number 1. *Arch Ophthalmol* 103:1796–1806, 1985

Ferris FL III, Davis MD, Aiello LM: Treatment of diabetic retinopathy. *N Engl J Med* 341:667–678, 1999

Ferris FL III: Results of 20 years of research on the treatment of diabetic retinopathy. *Prev Med* 23:740–742, 1994

Klein R: Prevention of visual loss from diabetic retinopathy. *Surv Ophthalmol* 47:S246–252, 2002

Klein R, Klein BE, Moss SE, Cruickshanks KJ: The Wisconsin epidemiology study of diabetic retinopathy. XIV. Ten-year incidence and progression of diabetic retinopathy. *Arch Ophthalmol* 112:1217–1228, 1994

Klein R, Klein BEK, Moss SE, Davis MD, DeMets DL: The Wisconsin epidemiology study of diabetic retinopathy. II. Prevalence and risk of diabetic retinopathy when age at diagnosis is less than 30 yr. *Arch Ophthalmol* 102:520–526, 1984

UK Prospective Diabetes Study Group: Intensive blood-glucose control with sulphonylureas or insulin compared with conventional treatment and risk of complications in patients with type 2 diabetes (UKPDS 33). *Lancet* 352:837–853, 1998

NEPHROPATHY

In the past, epidemiological studies have shown consistently that 20–30% of patients affected with type 1 diabetes will eventually develop end-stage renal failure and require dialysis. About 40% of individuals starting dialysis in the United States have diabetes, and almost half of these have type 1 diabetes. Evidence suggests that the frequency of nephropathy may be decreasing with the use of more effective diabetes treatment and antihypertensive therapy.

CLINICAL SYNDROME

In its fully established form, diabetic nephropathy is a distinct clinical entity characterized by proteinuria, hypertension, edema, and renal insufficiency; in its most severe forms, nephrotic syndrome can be present. Diabetic nephropathy occurs in type 1 diabetes patients with long-standing diabetes (usually >10 yr).

Histopathological Changes

Three classes of renal histopathological changes characterize diabetic nephropathy: *1)* glomerulosclerosis, *2)* structural vascular changes, particularly in the small arterioles, and *3)* tubulointerstitial disease. Glomerular damage, e.g., mesangial expansion and basement membrane thickening, is the most characteristic feature of diabetic nephropathy and most often takes the form of diffuse scarring of entire glomeruli. The tubulointerstitial changes interfere with potassium ion and hydrogen ion secretion and may be at least partly responsible for the hyperkalemia and metabolic acidosis that accompany diabetic renal disease.

NATURAL HISTORY

Shortly after diabetes is diagnosed, the glomerular filtration rate (GFR) and renal blood flow are characteristically elevated, and there is typically a corresponding increase in kidney weight and size. The increased GFR is related to the degree of hyperglycemia, and the GFR and renal hypertrophy can be normalized by improved glycemic control. The serum creatinine and urea nitrogen concentrations are slightly reduced when the renal hyperfiltration is present. Although a slight increase in urine protein is common when a patient initially presents in diabetic ketoacidosis, once glycemia is well regulated by insulin therapy, proteinuria disappears and remains absent for many years.

Early in the course of diabetes, the renal histology is normal despite renal hypertrophy. However, within 2–3 yr, many kidneys demonstrate some histological evidence of mesangial expansion and basement membrane thickening. Despite these histological changes, GFR and renal blood flow may remain elevated, and proteinuria is not detectable. The earliest clinical evidence of nephropathy is the appearance of low but abnormal levels (>30 mg/day or 20 µg/min) of albumin in the urine, referred to as microalbuminuria. Patients with microalbuminuria are referred to as having incipient nephropathy. This is a subclinical range of increased albumin excretion that goes undetected with routine urine testing. However, the development of more sensitive techniques has permitted the detection of these lower, yet abnormally elevated, albumin excretion rates. Microalbuminuria results vary widely from day to day, and abnormal results should be confirmed by repeat testing.

Patients with diabetes and microalbuminuria are at a higher risk for developing renal insufficiency and may benefit from more intensive follow-up and therapy. However, several factors can induce microalbuminuria, including poor glycemic control, stress, infection, and exercise. These must be excluded before drawing inferences from the presence of microalbuminuria. The presence of even microscopic hematuria is sufficient to invalidate tests for microalbuminuria. Therefore, measurements should not be made during menses or in the presence of urinary tract infection.

Without specific interventions, ~80% of subjects with type 1 diabetes who develop sustained microalbuminuria have their urinary albumin excretion increase at a rate of ~10–20%/yr to the stage of overt nephropathy or clinical albuminuria (>300 mg/24 h or ~200 µg/min) over 10–15 yr, with hypertension also developing. In addition to its being the earliest manifestation of nephropathy, microalbuminuria is a marker of greatly increased cardiovascular morbidity and mortality for patients with either type 1 or type 2 diabetes. Thus, the finding of microalbuminuria is an indication for screening for possible vascular disease and aggressive intervention to reduce all cardiovascular risk factors (e.g., lowering of LDL cholesterol, antihypertensive therapy, smoking cessation, increased physical activity). In addition, some preliminary evidence suggests that lowering cholesterol may also reduce the level of proteinuria.

Once overt nephropathy occurs, without specific interventions, the GFR gradually falls over several years at a rate that is highly variable from individual to individual (2–20 ml/min/yr). End-stage renal disease (ESRD) develops in 50% of patients with type 1 diabetes with overt nephropathy within 10 yr and in >75% by 20 yr.

Although the GFR may still be elevated at the onset of proteinuria, it usually declines by ~50% within 3 yr, and the serum creatinine and urea nitrogen concentrations become frankly elevated (>2.0 and >30 mg/dl, respectively). Within a mean of 2 yr after the serum creatinine becomes elevated (>2.0 mg/dl), 50% of the individuals will progress to end-stage renal failure. The mean duration of type 1 diabetes when ESRD develops is 23 yr. With ESRD, the uremic symptoms, e.g., drowsiness, lethargy, and nausea, appear and become progressively more pronounced. Most patients receive treatment before reaching this stage, and cardiovascular disease is now the most common cause of death in patients with nephropathy.

Traditionally, it has been considered unusual to observe diabetic nephropathy in the absence of retinopathy, neuropathy, and hypertension. However, the correlation is especially close only in advanced renal disease and is less common in type 2 diabetes. As kidney failure progresses, the incidence and severity of all three disorders increases markedly, generally in parallel with renal status.

PATHOGENESIS

Considerable evidence suggests that diabetic nephropathy is related primarily to the metabolic changes induced by the diabetic state. First, renal changes are absent initially in people biopsied around the time of onset of diabetes. Second, typical changes of diabetic nephropathy occur in all types of diabetes. Third, diabetic nephropathy appears in various animal models regardless of whether the diabetes is induced or spontaneous, and the damage occurs in both original and transplanted kidneys. Fourth, in these diabetic animals, intensive insulin therapy or islet cell transplantation completely prevents renal histopathologic changes and may reverse early histopathologic abnormalities. Last, improved glucose control can substantially delay the initial appearance of persistent microalbuminuria and clinical grade albuminuria in type 1 diabetes.

Possible Mechanisms of Damage

The mechanisms by which diabetes damages the kidney remain unknown. It has not been established whether elevated glucose per se or some metabolic event that occurs as a consequence of hyperglycemia is the trigger.

A genetic propensity to diabetic nephropathy also contributes to its development. Thus, it is possible that metabolic disturbances initiate the processes responsible for diabetic nephropathy but that these processes operate on a genetic background that predisposes to diabetic glomerulosclerosis. Some studies suggest the genetic predisposition relates to an increased familial incidence of essential hypertension.

One explanation for renal damage may involve the typical increases in GFR and renal blood flow that occur early in the course of diabetes. In animals, these alterations in renal hemodynamics are associated with increased intraglomerular pressures. Although it has not been possible to measure intraglomerular pressure in humans, it has been suggested that glomerular hypertension, regardless of what derangements or predispositions lead up to it, is the ultimate mediator of kidney damage in diabetic nephropathy. Measures aimed at reversing the resulting hemodynamic changes have proved useful in slowing the progression of renal disease in human diabetes.

MANAGEMENT

In the first 5 yr of diabetes, a routine urinalysis with a check for proteinuria should be obtained annually. Routine urinalysis should be performed yearly in adults. If positive for protein, a quantitative measure is frequently helpful in development of a treatment plan (see Table 6.2 for definitions of abnormalities). If the urinalysis is negative for protein, a test for the presence of microalbumin is necessary. Because microalbuminuria rarely occurs with short duration of type 1 diabetes or before puberty, screening in individuals with type 1 diabetes should begin with puberty and after disease duration of 5 yr. Evidence suggests that the prepubertal duration of diabetes may be important in the development of microvascular complications, so clinical judgment should be used when applying this recommendation to individual patients.

Screening for microalbuminuria can be performed by three methods: *1*) measurement of the albumin-to-creatinine ratio in a random spot collection, *2*) 24-h collection, and *3*) timed (e.g., 4-h or overnight) collection. The first method is often found to be the easiest to carry out in an office setting and generally pro-

Table 6.2 Definitions in Abnormalities of Albumin Excretion

Category	4-h Collection (mg/24 h)	Timed Collection (µg/min)	Spot Collection (µg/mg creatinine)
Normal	<30	<20	<30
Microalbuminuria	30–299	20–199	<30–299
Clinical albuminuria ≥300	≥200	≥300	

vides accurate information; first-void or other morning collections are preferred because of the known diurnal variation in albumin excretion, but if this timing cannot be used, uniformity of timing for different collections in the same individual should be employed. Specific assays are needed to detect microalbuminuria, because both standard dipsticks and standard hospital laboratory assays for urinary protein are not sufficiently sensitive to measure such levels. Microalbuminuria is defined as in Table 6.2. If assays for microalbuminuria are not readily available, screening with reagent tablets or dipsticks for microalbumin may be performed, because they show acceptable sensitivity (95%) and specificity (93%) when carried out by trained personnel. Because reagent strips only indicate concentration and do not correct for creatinine as the spot urine albumin-to-creatinine ratio does, they are subject to possible errors from alterations in urine concentration. All positive tests by reagent strips or tablets should be confirmed by more specific methods.

If microalbuminuria or proteinuria is present, serum creatinine and urea nitrogen concentrations should be measured and glomerular filtration assessed. Once microalbuminuria, overt proteinuria, or elevated serum creatinine or urea nitrogen is detected, renal function should be monitored at least two to three times per year. Consultation with a nephrologist is indicated to plot a long-term therapeutic strategy and to discuss the possibility and implications of renal failure with the patient.

Because of variability in urinary albumin excretion, at least two of three specimens collected within a 3- to 6-mo period should be abnormal before considering a patient to have crossed one of these diagnostic thresholds. Exercise within 24 h, infection, fever, congestive heart failure, marked hyperglycemia, and marked hypertension may elevate urinary albumin excretion over baseline values.

Hypertension should be aggressively treated. Otherwise, the management of diabetic nephropathy is largely preventive and supportive. It consists of *1)* minimizing factors that are known to accelerate the natural progression of renal disease or that may otherwise jeopardize the kidney and *2)* appropriately responding to changing insulin needs (Tables 6.3 and 6.4). If end-stage renal failure ensues, two options are available for renal replacement therapy: dialysis and kidney transplantation.

HYPERTENSION

In type 1 diabetes, hypertension typically is secondary to the onset of renal disease. Long-term survivors of diabetes without nephropathy rarely have hyper-

Table 6.3 Treatment of Diabetic Nephropathy

The following are factors influencing diabetic nephropathy and should be addressed:

- **Hypertension.** This is the most important factor shown to accelerate progression of renal failure. Goal blood pressure is <130 mmHg systolic and <80 mmHg diastolic. Angiotensin-converting enzyme (ACE) inhibitors and angiotensin II–receptor blockers (ARBs) have specific effects to preserve renal function.

- **Hyperglycemia.** Control of blood glucose is extremely important in preventing and stopping the progression of microalbuminuria and proteinuria. The recommended glycemic goals are as close to normal as possible (Table 2.1). Note that uremia may be associated with insulin resistance and increased insulin requirements. With advanced uremia (GFR 15–20 ml/min), insulin requirements may fall because the kidney removes 25% of daily injected insulin, and hepatic degradation of insulin is inhibited by uremia.

- **Hyperlipidemia.** Control of lipids (LDL <100 mg/dl) is essential in preventing cardiovascular disease and may aid in slowing the progression of nephropathy.

- **Proteinuria.** Reduction of proteinuria with ACE inhibitors, ARBs, and nondihydropyridine calcium antagonists have additive effects to preserve renal function.

- **Protein restriction.** A low-protein diet (<0.8 g/kg body wt/day) slows progression of renal disease in patients with diabetes with advanced renal insufficiency.

tension. Hypertension is also the single most important factor shown to accelerate the progression of established diabetic nephropathy and contributes to other causes of diabetes-related morbidity and mortality, e.g., retinopathy and heart disease. Both systolic and diastolic hypertension markedly accelerate the progression of diabetic nephropathy. Aggressive treatment of hypertension is the only therapeutic intervention definitively shown to slow the progression of established renal disease. It is paramount that blood pressure levels be controlled. Ideally, the patient with diabetes should have blood pressure normalized (<130/80 mmHg) to the extent possible without compromising cardiac, cerebral, or other organ-system functions. The minimal goal of therapy for nonpregnant patients with diabetes >18 yr of age is to decrease blood pressure to and maintain it at <130 mmHg systolic and <80 mmHg diastolic. For patients with isolated systolic hypertension with a systolic pressure of >180 mmHg, the initial goal of treatment is to reduce the systolic blood pressure in stages. If these initial goals are met and well tolerated, further lowering may be indicated.

Antihypertensive Therapy

The diagnosis of hypertension should be based on multiple blood pressure determinations before beginning treatment. Orthostatic hypotension is frequent in patients with diabetic nephropathy; therefore, both supine and standing blood pressure should be measured. Ambulatory blood pressure monitoring is used in some centers to monitor patients during treatment.

Angiotensin-converting enzyme (ACE) inhibitors. Many studies have shown that in hypertensive patients with type 1 diabetes, ACE inhibitors can reduce the

Table 6.4 Other Threats to Diabetic Kidneys

Several conditions can endanger the kidneys of individuals with diabetes, even if renal insufficiency has not yet come into play. Among them are the following:

- **Urinary tract infection.** Older individuals with diabetes generally have an increased incidence of urinary tract infection. Therefore, for these patients, it is important that a urinalysis be performed at each clinic visit. If leukocytes or bacteriuria are detected, a urine culture should be obtained. Positive cultures should be treated with an appropriate bactericidal antibiotic.
- **Neurogenic bladder.** The development of a neurogenic bladder is common in patients with diabetes, especially if other evidence of autonomic neuropathy is present, and may predispose to infection. Symptoms, e.g., frequent voiding, nocturia, incontinence, recurrent urinary tract infections, may be minimal or may mimic those of prostatic hypertrophy. Once suspected, the diagnosis is easily established if a cystometrogram demonstrates a large atonic bladder with low-pressure recordings. If the presence of a neurogenic bladder is confirmed, the patient should receive instruction in Credé's manual voiding maneuver, which should be performed every ~8 h. Often this will be sufficient to prevent postvoid residual and will decompress the upper urinary tract. If not, parasympathetic agents such as bethanechol chloride may be tried. In some people with diabetes, β-adrenergic–blocking agents, such as phenoxybenzamine, have proved useful. If pharmacologic therapy proves unsuccessful, intermittent straight catheterization should be performed 2–3 times daily.
- **Intravenous pyelography and other dye studies.** Patients with diabetes are at increased risk for acute renal failure after any radiocontrast (intravenous and retrograde pyelography, arteriography, cholangiography, computed tomography scanning) procedure. With the judicious use of echography, radionuclide studies, magnetic resonance imaging, and noncontrast computed tomography scanning, studies employing iodinated radiocontrast dye are rarely necessary. If contrast media must be used, a minimum amount of dye should be given, and adequate hydration with half-normal or normal saline should be ensured before the dye study. Use of iso-osmolar, dimeric, nonionic iodinated contrast agents such as iodixanol should be considered in high-risk patients with nephropathy or serum creatinine concentrations >1.5 mg/dl. General recommendations cannot yet be made regarding the routine administration of specific agents to prevent contrast-induced reductions in renal function, such as acetylcysteine or fenoldopam, as they are still under intensive investigation. Serum creatinine concentration should be checked daily for 2–3 days after the contrast study.

level of albuminuria and reduce the rate of progression of renal disease to a greater degree than other antihypertensive agents that lower blood pressure by an equal amount. These drugs even appear to be effective in patients with microalbuminuria with or without hypertension. ACE inhibitors are recommended as the primary treatment of all hypertensive type 1 diabetes patients with microalbuminuria or overt nephropathy. Because of the high proportion of patients who progress from microalbuminuria to overt nephropathy and subsequently to ESRD, use of ACE inhibitors is recommended for all type 1 diabetes patients with microalbuminuria, even if normotensive.

Results with captopril in patients with overt nephropathy have conclusively shown a beneficial effect on preserving kidney function. ACE inhibitors have few adverse effects and may even have modest beneficial effects on lipid metabolism and insulin sensitivity. The major serious side effect of ACE inhibitors is hyperkalemia, which is of particular concern in patients with more advanced nephropathy, who may have the syndrome of hyporeninemic hypoaldosteronism. In the presence of low renin, circulating aldosterone levels are decreased and the renal tubular secretion of potassium is impaired. Any drug that further impairs aldosterone secretion or action may lead to clinically significant hyperkalemia.

Some patients may experience a precipitous decline in renal function when initiating therapy with ACE inhibitors, especially those with bilateral renal artery stenosis or advanced renal disease, even without renal artery stenosis or decompensated congestive heart failure. Because this appears to be more common in patients with impaired renal function or renovascular hypertension, the physician should determine serum creatinine and potassium levels ~1 wk after therapy begins. An excessive increase in either level warrants discontinuation of the drug. Cough may also occur. Finally, ACE inhibitors are contraindicated in pregnancy and therefore should be used with caution in women of childbearing potential.

Angiotensin II–receptor blockers (ARBs). ARBs can slow the progression of renal disease. Studies have shown a slowing of the rate of transition from microalbuminuria to clinical albuminuria in hypertensive type 2 diabetes patients. Furthermore, in type 2 diabetes with hypertension, albuminuria, and elevated creatinine levels, ARBs clearly slow the progression of diabetic nephropathy compared with other antihypertensive agents. If ACE inhibitors cannot be tolerated because of side effects, such as cough, substitution of an ARB should be considered. Recent studies suggest that ARBs may be additive to ACE inhibitors in slowing the progression of diabetic nephropathy and decreasing proteinuria.

Diuretics. Because hypertension in the patient with diabetic nephropathy is often volume sensitive, therapy with a low-sodium diet and a diuretic when edema is present may be effective. Because many hypertensive individuals with diabetes have some degree of renal insufficiency, a loop diuretic is usually necessary. Thiazide diuretics do not promote diuresis once the serum creatinine level has risen to levels >1.5 mg/dl. When used, the dose of thiazide diuretics is lower than that used customarily. Hydrochlorothiazide, 12.5 or 25 mg daily, is as effective an antihypertensive and is better tolerated than larger doses. Potassium levels should be closely monitored, as hypokalemia may worsen glucose control. Also, use of diuretics that inhibit potassium secretion (e.g., spironolactone, triamterene) should be used with caution because of concern for inducing hyperkalemia.

β-Adrenergic–blocking agents. β-Adrenergic–blocking agents have also proven successful in treating the hypertensive patient with diabetes. However, this class of drugs inhibits hepatic glucose production, which may lead to hypoglycemia, and they may mask many of the warning symptoms of hypoglycemia (although sweating is not affected). β-Blocking agents also predispose the development of hyperkalemia by inhibiting renin synthesis and impairing potassium uptake by extrarenal tissues. Moreover, they aggravate any dyslipidemia that might be present. Specific β_1-antagonists are the preferred β-blocking agents in patients with diabetes because they are less likely to cause hypoglycemia and hyperkalemia.

Calcium antagonists. Studies have shown that nondihydropyridine calcium antagonists reduce microalbuminuria and proteinuria; however, the long-term renal-protective effects are unknown. This class of drugs is relatively free of harmful side effects and does not cause significant alterations in glucose or lipid metabolism.

OTHER ASPECTS OF TREATMENT

Blood Glucose Control

The DCCT demonstrated conclusively that intensive insulin therapy reduces the development and progression of early renal disease. An intensive treatment program is an essential component of the treatment of a patient found to have microalbuminuria. On the other hand, there is no evidence that tight glycemic control through intensive insulin therapy can reverse or even slow the progression of severely advanced renal disease.

The development of renal insufficiency is associated with insulin resistance, which may result in an increase in insulin requirements. However, because insulin is cleared by the kidney, as renal failure further worsens it is common to see a decrease in the daily insulin dose and/or an increase in hypoglycemic episodes, particularly in patients with a glomerular filtration rate <20 ml/min. For this reason, self-monitoring of blood glucose and use of the results to adjust the insulin dose are important.

Low-Protein Diet

Over the last several years, there has been renewed interest in the use of low-protein diets to prevent the progression of chronic renal failure (see Nutrition, page 85). Animal studies have shown that restriction of dietary protein intake also reduces hyperfiltration and intraglomerular pressure and retards the progression of several models of renal disease, including diabetic glomerulopathy. A meta-analysis of several small studies in humans with diabetic nephropathy indicated that protein-restricted diets reduce proteinuria and retard the rate of fall of GFR modestly. The general consensus is to prescribe a protein intake of approximately the adult recommended dietary allowance of 0.8 g/kg/day (~10% of daily calories) in patients with overt nephropathy. Once the GFR begins to fall, further restriction to 0.6 g/kg/day may prove useful in slowing the decline of GFR in selected patients.

A low-protein diet must be high in carbohydrate and/or fat; however, the long-term effects of such a diet on atherosclerotic complications and glycemic control are unknown. Nutrition deficiency may occur in some individuals and may be associated with muscle weakness. Similarly, it is not known whether a low-protein diet can maintain a normal nitrogen balance in a patient with diabetes with advanced renal insufficiency.

Low-protein diets are difficult for the patient to maintain, and a modest restriction in dietary protein combined with the other treatment measures may be more reasonable. Protein-restricted meal plans should be designed by a registered dietitian familiar with all components of the dietary management of diabetes.

DIALYSIS AND KIDNEY TRANSPLANTATION

Once ESRD progresses to renal failure, prolonging life requires dialysis or a functioning kidney transplant. A functioning kidney transplant provides the uremic patient with diabetes a greater survival with greater rehabilitation than does either continuous ambulatory peritoneal dialysis (CAPD) or maintenance hemodialysis. No matter which ESRD therapy has been elected, optimal rehabilitation in ESRD patients requires that effort be devoted to recognition and management of comorbid conditions. Uremia therapy, whether CAPD, hemodialysis, or a kidney transplant, should be individualized to the patient's specific medical and family circumstances. The pros and cons of these procedures should be discussed with patients and their families well in advance of end-stage renal failure. The prospect of needing such measures should never be a surprise. The ultimate choice among alternatives requires input from the patient, the patient's family, a nephrologist, and the primary care physician. In patients with diabetes, the absolute indications for dialysis or transplantation occur earlier than with other causes of ESRD, i.e., at serum creatinine >6 mg/dl or creatinine clearance ≤20 ml/min, as well as urgent uremic symptoms, e.g., seizures, uremic pericarditis, unresponsive hypertension, and muscle deterioration. More subjective criteria include worsening lethargy, nausea or vomiting, and progressive retinopathy and neuropathy. It is important not to delay the start of dialysis in patients with diabetes.

Renal Dialysis

Of the various forms of renal dialysis, hemodialysis is the most frequently used in patients with diabetes, although types of peritoneal dialysis have also been used with success. Some patients using peritoneal dialysis have insulin included with the dialysate. This procedure often improves blood glucose control because peritoneal insulin delivery is more physiologic than subcutaneous delivery. Peritoneal dialysis also affords a motivated patient the greatest mobility. Treatment of anemia with erythropoietin has substantially improved the general well-being both of patients on dialysis and of patients before the initiation of dialysis therapy.

Kidney Transplantation

When the success rate of kidney transplantation in patients with diabetes approached the excellent success rate achieved in patients without diabetes, this procedure became the treatment of choice in patients with diabetic ESRD. Kidneys donated by first-degree relatives continue to be preferable, although increasing experience with immunosuppressive agents has helped lower the incidence of rejection with cadaver-donated kidneys. Transplantation from a living unrelated donor, such as a spouse or close friend, is a highly successful procedure that is being used more commonly.

The decision of whether to opt for a transplant is still not one to be taken lightly, and a patient must be well briefed on the chances of failure, as well as the possibility that the new kidney will undergo the same changes that caused the original kidneys to fail. This risk means that the patient should be considered for initiation of an intensive insulin treatment program posttransplantation. Serious consideration should be devoted to a combined kidney and pancreas transplant to control hyperglycemia in type 1 diabetes patients, which can often be successfully performed. Combination transplantation increases short-term morbidity, but properly selected patients may have better long-term rehabilitation.

CONCLUSION

ESRD is a major cause of morbidity and mortality in patients with type 1 diabetes of >15 yr duration. Vigilant monitoring of evolving proteinuria and in particular its early detection with microalbuminuria testing, striving for excellent glycemic control within patient-acceptable goals, aggressive therapy of hypertension, and anticipating the need for dialysis or transplantation form the cornerstones of management. The primary care provider is pivotal in integrating available resources, including referral to a nephrologist. The options available in the event of end-stage renal failure offer greater possibilities than were available even 5 yr ago for salvaging quality of life and increasing longevity. When possible, renal transplantation is advised as the treatment most likely to effect rehabilitation and long survival.

BIBLIOGRAPHY

American Diabetes Association: Diabetic nephropathy (Position Statement). *Diabetes Care* 26 (Suppl. 1):S94–S98, 2003

American Diabetes Association: Treatment of hypertension in adults with diabetes (Position Statement). *Diabetes Care* 26 (Suppl. 1):S80–S82, 2003

Aspelin P, Aubry P, Fransson S-G, Strasser R, Willenbrock R, Berg KJ, Nephrotoxicity in High-Risk Patients Study of Iso-Osmolar and Low-Osmolar Non-Ionic Contrast Media Study Investigators: Nephrotoxic effects in high-risk patients undergoing angiography. *N Engl J Med* 348:491–499, 2003

Bennett PH, Haffner S, Kasiske BL, Keane WF, Mogensen CE, Parving H-H, Steffes MW, Striker GE: Screening and management of microalbuminuria in patients with diabetes mellitus. *Am J Kidney Dis* 25:107–112, 1995

Brenner BM, Cooper ME, de Zeeuw D, Keane WF, Mitch WE, Parving H-H, Remuzzi G, Snapinn SM, Zhang Z, Shahinfar S, for the RENAAL study investigators: Effects of losartan on renal and cardiovascular outcomes in patients with type 2 diabetes and nephropathy. *N Engl J Med* 345:861–869, 2001

DCCT Research Group: The effect of intensive treatment of diabetes on the development and progression of long-term complications in insulin-dependent diabetes mellitus. *N Engl J Med* 329:977–986, 1993

Jacobson HR, Striker GE, for the Workshop Group: Report on a workshop to develop management recommendations for the prevention of progression in chronic renal disease. *Am J Kidney Dis* 25:103–106, 1995

Kasiske BL, Kalil RSN, Ma JZ, Liao M, Keane WF: Effect of antihypertensive therapy on the kidney in patients with diabetes: a meta-regression analysis. *Ann Intern Med* 118:129–138, 1993

Kopple JD, Hakim RM, Held PJ, Keane WF, King K, Lazarus JM, Parker TF, Teehan BP: National Kidney Foundation: Recommendations for reducing the high morbidity and mortality of U.S. maintenance hemodialysis patients (Position Paper). *Am J Kidney Dis* 24:968–973, 1994

Krolewski AS, Warram JH: Natural history of diabetic nephropathy. *Diabetes Reviews* 3:446–459, 1995

La Rocca E, Fiorina P, di Carlo V, Astorri E, Rossetti C, Lucignani G, Fazio F, Giudici D, Cristallo M, Bianchi G, Pozza G, Secchi A: Cardiovascular outcomes after kidney-pancreas and kidney-alone transplantation. *Kidney Int* 60:1964–1971, 2001

Lewis JL, Hunsicker LG, Bain RP: The effect of angiotensin-converting enzyme inhibition on diabetic nephropathy. *N Engl J Med* 329:1456–1462, 1993

Manske CL: Hyperglycemia and intensive glycemic control in diabetic patients with chronic renal disease. *Am J Kidney Dis* 32:S157–S171, 1998

Microalbuminuria Captopril Study Group: Captopril reduces the risk of nephropathy in IDDM patients with microalbuminuria. *Diabetologia* 39:587–593, 1996

Mogensen CE, Christensen CK: Predicting diabetic nephropathy in insulin-dependent patients. *N Engl J Med* 311:89–93, 1984

Mogensen CE, Keane WF, Bennett PH, Jerums G, Parving H-H, Passa P, Steffes MW, Striker GE, Viberti GC: Prevention of diabetic renal disease with special reference to microalbuminuria. *Lancet* 346:1080–1084, 1995

Pedrini MT, Levey AS, Lau J, Chalmers TC, Wang PH: The effect of dietary protein restriction on the progression of diabetic and nondiabetic renal diseases: a meta-analysis. *Ann Intern Med* 124:627–632, 1996

Remuzzi G, Ruggenenti P, Perico N: Chronic renal diseases: renoprotective benefits of renin-angiotensin system inhibition. *Ann Intern Med* 136:604–615, 2002

Ritz E, Rychlík I, Locatelli F, Halimi S: End-stage renal failure in type 2 diabetes: a medical catastrophe of worldwide dimensions. *Am J Kidney Dis* 34:795–808, 1999

Viberti GC, Wiseman MJ: The kidney in diabetes: significance of the early abnormalities. *Clin Endocrinol Metab* 15:753–782, 1986

Zatz R, Brenner BM: Pathogenesis of diabetic microangiopathy: the hemodynamic view. *Am J Med* 80:443–453, 1986

NEUROPATHY

Peripheral neuropathy is one of the most common and troubling chronic complications of diabetes. Virtually all regions of the body can be affected by diabetic neuropathy, which can produce significant impairments alone and in concert with other conditions. Most notably, neuropathic loss of sensation in the foot regularly conspires with infection and/or vascular insufficiency (more common in people with diabetes) to make diabetes the most frequent source of nontraumatic lower-limb amputations in the United States.

OVERVIEW OF NEUROPATHIES

The frequency of diabetic neuropathy parallels duration and severity of hyperglycemia in both type 1 and type 2 diabetes. In patients with type 1 diabetes, it rarely occurs within the first 5 yr after diagnosis. Sometimes the symptoms become manifest only after the initiation of insulin therapy. Neuropathy in diabetes can also be caused by pancreatectomy, nonalcoholic pancreatitis, and hemochromatosis, as well as independently in conditions more commonly associated with type 1 diabetes, e.g., hypothyroidism and pernicious anemia.

Histological Findings

Histologically, there is loss of both large and small myelinated nerve fibers, accompanied by varying degrees of paranodal and segmental demyelination, connective tissue proliferation, and thickening and reduplication of capillary basement membranes with capillary closure. Researchers are investigating several potential pathways by which hyperglycemia (perhaps aided by other metabolic derangements of diabetes) may cause such changes. The polyol pathway, protein glycation, and altered intracellular oxidation-reduction potential are prominent among the mechanisms being studied.

Treatment of Neuropathies

There is no known direct treatment for neuropathy. The DCCT demonstrated that intensive treatment programs reduce by 60% the development and progression of early neuropathy. Aldose reductase inhibitors (ARIs) block the rate-limiting enzyme in the polyol pathway, which is activated in hyperglycemic states. ARIs, α-lipoic acid, nerve growth factor, glycation reaction inhibitors, and γ-linolenic acid have been shown to improve nerve conduction in diabetic animals and patients with diabetes. However, results in clinical trials in symptomatic neuropathy have been negative or have shown only modest effectiveness in more advanced forms of neuropathy. Studies with α-lipoic acid and protein kinase C inhibitor are ongoing.

Clinical Syndrome

Diabetic neuropathy is classified into a set of discrete clinical syndromes, each with a characteristic presentation and clinical course (Table 6.5). Because the syndromes overlap clinically and frequently occur simultaneously, rigid classification of individual cases is often difficult. Identical neurological syndromes occur

Table 6.5 Syndromes of Diabetic Neuropathy

Diffuse neuropathies (common, insidious onset, usually progressive)	■ Cranial neuropathy
	■ Radiculopathy
■ Distal symmetrical sensorimotor polyneuropathy	■ Plexopathy
	■ Mononeuropathy/mononeuropathy multiplex
■ Autonomic neuropathy	
Focal neuropathies (sudden onset, usually improve over time)	■ Other mononeuropathies

in other diseases and other conditions. For example, alcoholic neuropathy and inflammatory neuropathies can mimic peripheral diabetic neuropathy. Diabetic neuropathy is a diagnosis of exclusion (Table 6.6).

DISTAL SYMMETRIC SENSORIMOTOR POLYNEUROPATHY

Distal symmetric polyneuropathy is the most common form of diabetic neuropathy. Sensory signs and symptoms generally predominate over motor involvement and vary depending on the classes of nerve fibers. Loss of large fibers produces diminished proprioception and light touch, resulting in ataxic gait, unsteadiness, and weakness of intrinsic muscles in the hands and feet. Involvement of small fibers causes diminished pain and temperature sensation, resulting in unrecognized trauma (especially to the feet), accidental burning of the hands, etc.

Typical neuropathic paresthesia (spontaneous uncomfortable sensations) or dysesthesia (contact paresthesia) may accompany both large- and small-fiber involvement. Sensory deficits first appear in the most distal portions of the extremities and spread proximally with disease progression in a "stocking-glove" distribution. In the most advanced cases, vertical bands of sensory deficit develop on the chest or abdomen when the tips of the shorter truncal nerves become involved (Fig. 6.9).

Occasionally, patients complain of exquisite hypersensitivity to light touch, superficial burning or stabbing pain, or bone-deep aching or tearing pain, usually most troublesome at night. Sometimes, neuropathic pain may become the overriding and disabling feature, especially in small-fiber neuropathy. Both neuropathic pain and paresthesia are thought to reflect spontaneous depolarization of newly regenerating nerve fibers.

Asymptomatic Neuropathy

Many patients with distal symmetrical polyneuropathy remain free of troubling, subjective symptoms. In these cases, it may take careful questioning to learn of a patient's subtle feelings of numbness or cold or "dead" feet. Diminished or absent deep-tendon reflexes, especially the Achilles tendon reflex, is often an early indication of otherwise asymptomatic neuropathy. However, in the absence of pain or paresthesia, diabetic neuropathy may go unrecognized unless the physician routinely tests foot sensation during office visits.

Table 6.6 Common Conditions Resembling Various Forms of Diabetic Neuropathy

Distal symmetrical neuropathy

- Inflammatory neuropathies (vasculitic, i.e., systemic lupus erythematosus, polyarteritis, and other connective tissue diseases; sarcoidosis; leprosy)
- Metabolic neuropathies (hypothyroidism, uremic; nutritional; acute intermittent porphyria)
- Toxic neuropathies (alcohol; drugs; heavy metals, e.g., lead, mercury, and arsenic; industrial hydrocarbons)
- Other neuropathies (paraneoplastic; dysproteinemic, amyloid, hereditary)

Autonomic neuropathy

- Pure autonomic failure (idiopathic orthostatic hypotension, Bradbury-Eggleston syndrome)
- Autoimmune autonomic neuropathy

Cranial neuropathy

- Carotid aneurysm
- Intracranial mass
- Elevated intracranial pressure

Radiculopathy

- Spinal cord/root compression
- Transverse myelitis
- Coagulopathies
- Shingles

Plexopathy

- Mass lesions
- Coagulopathies
- Cauda equina lesions (femoral neuropathy)

Mononeuropathy/mononeuropathy multiplex

- Compression neuropathies
- Inflammatory (vasculitic) neuropathies
- Hypothyroidism, acromegaly

LATE COMPLICATIONS OF POLYNEUROPATHY

Patients with chronic unrecognized neuropathy may present with late complications, e.g., foot ulceration, foreign objects embedded in the foot, unrecognized trauma to the extremities, or neuroarthropathy (Charcot's joints). All of these conditions are avoidable with proper early diagnosis of neuropathy and institution of appropriate foot care.

Foot Ulcerations and Infections

Acute foot ulcerations and resulting infections can occur when an individual cannot feel the pain caused by poorly fitting shoes (a source of penetrating abrasions), a retained foreign body, or accidental trauma (often unintentionally self-inflicted during nail trimming) because of neuropathy. Plantar ulcers, which form at the calloused sites of maximal walking pressure, can result from a combination of motor, sensory, and proprioceptive deficits.

Patients with long-standing diabetes and neuropathy are also predisposed to vascular ulcers due to macrovascular and microvascular insufficiency and ischemic gangrene.

In a typical sequence of events, imbalance of extensor and flexor muscles in the feet, resulting from impaired proprioception and atrophy of intrinsic extensor muscles, leads to tendon shortening and chronic toe flexion (claw toe or ham-

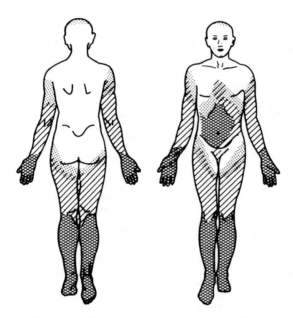

Figure 6.9 Distribution of sensory loss in patient with severe chronic diabetic sensory polyneuropathy. Loss is maximal distally in limbs but also affects anterior trunk and vertex of head. Hatched lines, pinprick impaired; crosshatched lines, pinprick absent; stippled lines, hyperesthesia. From Sabin TD, Geschwind M, Waxman SG: Patterns of clinical deficits in peripheral nerve disease. In *Physiology and Pathophysiology of Axons.* New York, Raven, 1987, p. 431–438.

mertoe deformity). This, in turn, shifts weight bearing from the padded ball of the foot to the unprotected metatarsal heads. With pain insensitivity, trauma to the overlying skin goes undetected, producing thick calluses that further concentrate weight bearing over the bony prominences. Splitting and fissuring of the thick callus or underlying pressure necrosis initiates ulcer formation, further aggravated by infection and vascular insufficiency.

Neuroarthropathy

Neuroarthropathy refers to the joint erosions, unrecognized fractures, demineralization, and devitalization of bones in the foot resulting from ignoring the minor injuries that occur during routine daily weight-bearing activities. Neuropathy impairs normal protective proprioceptive and nociceptive functions, which should lead the patient to recognize the injury and protect the foot. The foot may be swollen and red, but it is not painful. The problem may be misdiagnosed as cellulitis despite a normal leukocyte count and differential and the absence of fever. The patient may report relatively painless trauma, and initial radiographic examination may be unrevealing, whereas follow-up X rays several days or weeks later may reveal clear traumatic changes. In more advanced cases, devitalization of bone may mimic osteomyelitis, and in the most advanced stages, the foot may look like a "bag of bones."

MANAGEMENT OF DISTAL SYMMETRIC POLYNEUROPATHY AND COMPLICATIONS

Treatment for diabetic distal symmetric polyneuropathy is symptomatic, palliative, and supportive, with primary emphasis on preventing the neuropathy and vasculopathy by near-normalization of glucose and lipids and smoking cessation. In most cases, the primary neuropathic symptoms consist of mild intermittent pain or paresthesia. Even severely painful symptoms generally remit spontaneously within a few months in most but not all patients.

Management of Pain

Persistent and severely painful neuropathy has been treated with various drugs, including standard analgesics and drugs normally used to treat pain in other conditions. Narcotics should generally be avoided. The tricyclic drugs are the first-line drugs for the relief of painful neuropathic symptoms. Their efficacy, which has been proven in controlled trials, is related to plasma drug levels, and the onset of symptomatic relief is faster than their antidepressive effects. Numerous other drug therapies, including most antidepressants, have been reported to be useful in the relief of painful or paresthetic neuropathic symptoms. The anticonvulsant gabapentin is the best validated of the anticonvulsants used to treat painful neuropathy. Carbamazepine, oxcarbazepine, lamotrigine, zonisamide, topiramate, and phenytoin have been used based on their membrane-stabilizing properties. The antiarrhythmic drugs mexiletine and lidocaine may have similar effectiveness. Topical capsaicin applied frequently to the hypersensitive areas may be useful in some cases, especially those with more localized pain. Transcutaneous electrical nerve stimulation has also been used for refractory painful neuropathy. Other physical therapy measures, such as contrast baths and stretching exercises, provide ancillary help. Traditional therapies, such as acupuncture, have also been employed in painful neuropathy.

Because early diagnosis of asymptomatic neuropathy is essential for preventing the late complications, every routine physician visit should include a thorough examination of the feet if the patient has preexisting risk factors or any foot symptoms. A list of neurologic and related symptoms to watch for is given in Table 6.7.

Callus Formation and Plantar Ulcers

Callus formation over weight-bearing areas indicates the need to consult an orthopedist and/or podiatrist for prescription of corrective footwear to redistribute weight bearing. Plantar ulcers should be managed by eliminating weight bearing either by special walking casts or by bed rest. Local debridement and application of growth factors may speed healing. Refractory and/or recurrent ulcers may be managed by surgical removal of the involved metatarsal. If there is evidence of impaired macrovascular circulation, vascular studies should be

Table 6.7 Warning Symptoms and Signs of Diabetic Foot Problems

Symptoms

Vascular	Cold feet
	Intermittent claudication involving calf or foot
	Pain at rest, especially nocturnal, relieved by dependency
Neurologic	Sensory: burning, tingling, or crawling sensations; pain and hypersensitivity; complaints of cold or "dead" feet
	Motor weakness (drop foot)
	Autonomic: diminished sweating
Musculoskeletal	Gradual change in foot shape
	Sudden painless change in foot shape, with swelling, without history of trauma
Dermatologic	Exquisitely painful or painless wounds
	Slow-healing or nonhealing wounds, necrosis
	Skin color changes (cyanosis, redness)
	Chronic scaling, cracking, itching, or dry feet
	Recurrent infections (e.g., paronychia, athlete's foot)

Signs

Absent pedal, popliteal, or femoral pulses

Femoral bruits

Dependent rubor, plantar pallor on elevation

Prolonged capillary filling time (>3–4 s)

Decreased skin temperature

Sensory: deficits (vibratory and proprio perceptive, then pain and temperature perception), hyperesthesia

Motor: diminished to absent deep-tendon reflexes (Achilles then patellar), weakness

Autonomic: diminished to absent sweating

Cavus feet with claw toes

Drop foot

"Rockerbottom" foot (Charcot's joint)

Neuropathic arthropathy

Skin
- Abnormal dryness
- Chronic tinea infections
- Keratotic lesions with or without hemorrhage (plantar or digital)
- Trophic ulcer

Hair
- Diminished to absent

Nails
- Trophic changes
- Onychomycosis
- Subungual ulceration or abscess
- Ingrown nails with paronychia

From Scardina RJ: Diabetic foot problems: assessment and prevention. *Clinical Diabetes* 1:1–7, 1983.

obtained and revascularization attempted when indicated. Neuroarthropathy is managed by reduced ambulation and weight bearing, as well as cushioned footwear.

Treatment of Infection

Infection must be treated aggressively with appropriate consultation from infectious disease specialists. Antibiotics effective against aerobic and anaerobic organisms should be included in the treatment regimen. Deep-wound cultures are necessary to direct antibiotic therapy properly. Vascular bypass surgery or percutaneous angioplasty should be considered if arterial insufficiency is a major contributing factor. Localized osteomyelitis may require a limited amputation. Hyperbaric oxygen therapy may be indicated in refractory cases with impaired oxygenation of the surrounding tissue.

AUTONOMIC NEUROPATHY

Neuropathy can affect virtually any autonomic function in patients with diabetes. Although autonomic neuropathy produces diffuse subclinical dysfunction, autonomic symptoms are usually confined to one or two organ systems, producing the discrete autonomic syndromes listed in Table 6.8.

Cardiovascular Autonomic Neuropathy

The earliest clinical signs of cardiovascular autonomic neuropathy are absence of the normal sleep bradycardia and diminished variation of the pulse rate with inspiration-expiration or Valsalva (reduced sinus tachycardia), both due to early vagal involvement.

Table 6.8 Syndromes of Autonomic Neuropathy

Cardiovascular Autonomic Neuropathy	Genitourinary Autonomic Neuropathy
▪ Resting sinus tachycardia without sinus arrhythmia (fixed heart rate)	▪ Erectile dysfunction
▪ Exercise intolerance	▪ Retrograde ejaculation with infertility
▪ Painless myocardial infarction	▪ Bladder dysfunction
▪ Orthostatic hypotension	**Hypoglycemia Unawareness**
▪ Sudden death	**Sudomotor Neuropathy**
Gastrointestinal Autonomic Neuropathy	▪ Distal hyperhidrosis or anhidrosis
▪ Esophageal dysfunction	▪ Facial sweating
▪ Autonomic gastropathy and delayed gastric emptying	▪ Heat intolerance
▪ Diabetic diarrhea	▪ "Gustatory" sweating
▪ Constipation	
▪ Fecal incontinence	
▪ Gallbladder atony	

Later, sympathetic denervation interferes with normal cardiovascular reflexes thereby diminishing exercise tolerance, possibly hypersensitizing the heart to circulating catecholamines, tachyarrhythmias, and sudden death. It also predisposes to painless myocardial infarction.

Orthostatic hypotension. Orthostatic hypotension is managed by correcting hypovolemia with fluid replacement and improved diabetes control, elastic stockings, increased salt intake, mineralocorticoids, or vasoconstrictors. Midodrine, a specific α_1-agonist, has been shown to produce arteriolar constriction and decrease in venous pooling via a constriction of venous capacitance vessels.

Gastrointestinal (GI) Autonomic Neuropathy

Nonspecific GI symptoms in patients with diabetes often reflect diffuse but subtle GI autonomic dysfunction. Esophageal dysmotility can cause dysphagia, retrosternal discomfort, and heartburn. Delayed gastric emptying (gastroparesis) causes anorexia, nausea, vomiting, early satiety, and postprandial bloating and fullness. Delayed nutrient absorption can greatly complicate glycemic control, producing otherwise unexplained swings between severe hyperglycemia and hypoglycemia. Diagnosis of upper GI symptoms requires liquid and solid-phase radionuclide gastric-emptying studies. Management of esophageal dysmotility and delayed gastric emptying includes normalization of glucose and frequent small and/or primarily liquid feedings. High-fiber diets should be avoided, because they delay gastric emptying and may result in bezoar formation. Dopamine antagonists, such as metoclopramide or domperidone, may be helpful. Refractory cases may need gastric pacing or a feeding jejunostomy.

Diabetic constipation is the most frequent GI complaint, occurring in 60% of patients with diabetes. Stool softeners and laxatives or cathartics used judiciously are usually effective, although dopamine antagonists are occasionally indicated. Tegaserod maleate, an agonist of 5-HT$_4$ neurotransmitter in the GI tract, has been approved in treating constipation with additional relief of abdominal pain and bloating in female patients with irritable bowel syndrome. Studies are ongoing using this serotonin agonist in treating constipation and gastroparesis in patients with diabetes.

Diabetic diarrhea is classically painless, nocturnal, associated with fecal incontinence, and alternates with periods of constipation. Diagnostic studies of lower GI problems are necessary to define the multiple contributing factors that stem from widespread intestinal autonomic dysfunction to determine appropriate treatment. A therapeutic trial of broad-spectrum antibiotics may also be helpful, whereas evidence of bile salt malabsorption would argue in favor of bile salt–sequestering agents, both of which are effective in properly selected patients. Hypermotility is managed with diphenoxylate hydrochloride.

Fecal incontinence, which is also usually nocturnal, reflects impaired sensation of rectal distention, and in one small series of patients, it was effectively managed with biofeedback techniques. Clonidine has also been found useful.

Sexual Dysfunction

Erectile dysfunction. Erectile dysfunction in men with diabetes is usually neuropathic but can also be psychogenic, endocrine, vascular, or drug or stress related.

A normal erection on awakening or impotence only with a certain partner suggests a psychogenic cause. A band-type turgidity gauge or nocturnal penile tumescence monitoring at a sleep research facility can help clarify ambiguous situations.

Sex steroid imbalances, hypogonadotrophism, and hyperprolactinemia should be excluded by appropriate endocrine studies. Proximal vascular insufficiency is usually evident on examination of the femoral pulses, although localized obstruction of the penile artery has been reported and can be excluded only by measurement of the brachial-penile blood pressure ratio with Doppler-flow studies. Proximal or localized vascular obstruction has been managed surgically, but the success rate is low.

Drugs known to produce impotence include various antihypertensives, anticholinergics, antipsychotics, antidepressants, narcotics, barbiturates, alcohol, and amphetamines. Drug-induced impotence is managed by altering the treatment regimen when possible. Neuropathic impotence is generally but not always accompanied by other manifestations of diabetic neuropathy. Neuropathic impotence may be managed by appropriate counseling and penile prostheses when indicated.

The main therapy for erectile impotence of nonvascular or nonpsychological etiology has been the oral agent sildenafil. Sildenafil is a potent and competitive inhibitor of type 5 c-GMP-specific phosphodiesterase enzyme, the predominant isoenzyme in human corpus cavernosum. Very encouraging results have been presented for the oral agent sildenafil in the treatment of erectile dysfunction of diverse causes, including diabetes. The intracorporeal injection of vasoactive substances such as papaverine and prostaglandins are also effective in treating nonvascular erectile dysfunction.

Retrograde ejaculation. Retrograde ejaculation, which may or may not occur in conjunction with impotence, reflects loss of the coordinated closure of the internal and relaxation of the external vesicle sphincter during ejaculation. Presentation is usually infertility, and diagnosis is confirmed by documenting ejaculate azoospermia and the presence of motile sperm in postcoital urine. Such sperm have been successfully used for artificial insemination.

Other Autonomic Syndromes

Diabetic cystopathy. Cystopathy initially diminishes sensation of bladder fullness, reducing urinary frequency. Later, efferent involvement produces incomplete urination, poor stream, dribbling, and overflow incontinence, and it predisposes to urinary tract infections.

Conservative management involves scheduled voluntary urination with or without Credé's maneuver. Cholinergic-stimulating drugs, sphincter relaxants, periodic catheterization, and bladder-neck resection of the internal sphincter may be used in more advanced cases.

Hypoglycemia unawareness. Hypoglycemia unawareness may be related to autonomic neuropathy, which can blunt the usual adrenergic response to hypoglycemia. This is generally conceded to predispose to severe hypoglycemia. Increasing the lower glycemic target and use of insulin pump therapy is often needed to minimize or prevent recurrent spells of severe hypoglycemia.

Autonomic sudomotor dysfunction. Autonomic sudomotor dysfunction produces an asymptomatic anhydrosis of the extremities and compensatory central hyperhidrosis. It diminishes thermoregulatory reserve and predisposes to heat stroke and hyperthermia. Management is confined to avoidance of heat stress. The first specific treatment for diabetic gustatory sweating is glycopyrrolate, an antimuscarinic compound, which, when applied topically to the affected area, results in a marked reduction in sweating while eating a meal.

FOCAL NEUROPATHIES

Neural deficits corresponding to the distribution of single or multiple peripheral nerves (mononeuropathy and mononeuropathy multiplex), cranial nerves, areas of the brachial or lumbosacral plexuses (plexopathy), or the nerve roots (radiculopathy) are of sudden onset and generally but not always self-limiting in patients with diabetes.

The third cranial nerve may be affected, presenting with unilateral pain, diplopia, and ptosis but with pupillary sparing. Differential diagnosis includes an aneurysm of the internal carotid artery and myasthenia gravis. Spontaneous remission usually occurs within a few months.

Radiculopathy presents as band-like thoracic or abdominal pain, often misdiagnosed as an acute intrathoracic or intra-abdominal emergency.

Femoral neuropathy in patients with diabetes often involves motor and sensory deficits at the level of the sacral plexus as well as the femoral nerve, with the relative excess of motor versus sensory involvement differentiating diabetic femoral neuropathy from that seen in other conditions. When bilateral, this is sometimes termed amyotrophy. Management of focal neuropathies includes exclusion of other causes, e.g., nerve entrapment or compression and symptomatic palliation pending spontaneous resolution, which occurs generally but not always over periods of months to years.

CONCLUSION

Diabetic neuropathy is an extremely common complication of diabetes that becomes more prevalent with increasing duration and severity of hyperglycemia. Manifestations include diffuse and focal painful and painless neurological deficits in the peripheral nervous system and widespread autonomic dysfunction. Prompt and proper diagnosis is essential to effective management and avoidance of serious secondary musculoskeletal and visceral complications.

BIBLIOGRAPHY

American Diabetes Association: Preventive foot care in people with diabetes (Position Statement). *Diabetes Care* 26 (Suppl. 1):S78–S79, 2003

Backonja MM: Use of anticonvulsants for treatment of neuropathic pain. *Neurology* 59 (Suppl. 2):S14–S17, 2002

DCCT Research Group: The effect of intensive treatment of diabetes on the development and progression of long-term complications in insulin-dependent diabetes mellitus. *N Engl J Med* 329:977–986, 1993

Dyck PJ, Thomas PK, Asbury AK, Winegrad AI, Porte D (Eds.): *Diabetic Neuropathy*. Philadelphia, PA, WB Saunders, 1987

Gries FA, Cameron NE, Low PA, Ziegler D (Eds): *Textbook of Diabetic Neuropathy*. New York, Thieme, 2003

Low PA (Ed): *Clinical Autonomic Disorders: Evaluation and Management*. 2nd ed. Philadelphia, PA, Lippincott-Raven, 1997

Low PA, Dotson RM: Symptomatic treatment of painful neuropathy (Editorial). *JAMA* 280:1863–1864, 1998

Maser RE, Mitchell BD, Vinik AI, Freeman R: The association between cardiovascular autonomic neuropathy and mortality in individuals with diabetes: a meta-analysis. *Diabetes Care* 26:1895–1901, 2003

Parry GJ: Management of diabetic neuropathy. *Am J Med* 107:27S–33S, 1999

Simmons Z, Feldman EL: Update on diabetic neuropathy. *Curr Opin Neurol* 15:595–603, 2002

Vinik AI, Maser RE, Mitchell BD, Freeman R: Diabetic autonomic neuropathy. *Diabetes Care* 26:1553–1579, 2003

Vinik AI, Park TS, Stansberry KB, Pittenger GL: Diabetic neuropathies. *Diabetologia* 43:957–973, 2000

MACROVASCULAR DISEASE

Coronary heart disease, peripheral arterial disease, and cerebrovascular disease all occur more commonly, at an earlier age, with a more diffuse distribution and with greater severity and mortality in people with diabetes compared to patients without diabetes. Diabetes itself has been elevated in status from a risk factor for cardiovascular disease, to a coronary heart disease (CHD) risk equivalent in the National Cholesterol Education Panel Adult Treatment Program III (NCEP ATP III) guidelines. These guidelines focus on the necessity of aggressive preventive strategies for all patients with diabetes.

The NCEP ATP III recommendations are to be applied to patients with type 2 diabetes at the time of diagnosis. At this time, there is no consensus on the appropriate patient age or duration of type 1 diabetes that signals the need for aggressive preventive steps. This decision is left to the individual health care provider. In patients without diabetes, men age >45 yr and women age >55 yr are considered to be at increased risk for CHD. Certainly, patients with type 1 diabetes should receive preventive therapies, beyond good glycemic control, at ages younger than these gender-based thresholds. Although the prevalence of hypercholesterolemia is the same in patients with and without type 1 diabetes, the high absolute risk of heart disease in patients with type 1 diabetes creates an opportunity of substantial benefit to prevent events when lipid treatment guidelines are followed. Other risk factors, including hypertension, which is more prevalent in people with type 1 diabetes than in the general population, as well as cigarette smoking, which is as common among people with diabetes as in the general population, must also receive attention.

PREVALENCE AND RISK FACTORS

Although cardiovascular deaths are less common in patients with type 1 diabetes than in generally older patients with type 2 diabetes, mortality rates among individuals with type 1 diabetes are excessive. Patients with type 1 diabetes have an at least 10-fold increase in mortality compared to individuals of the same age without diabetes. Overall, atherosclerotic cardiovascular disease (ASCVD) accounts for ~25% of the deaths among patients with the onset of diabetes before age 20 yr. Premature CHD and stroke cause 27% and 6%, respectively, of the deaths among patients with diabetes age <45 yr. Many of these deaths occur in patients with diabetic nephropathy, and a large percentage of them result from the unfavorable and avoidable interactions of diabetes, hypertension, and cigarette smoking.

Diabetes is an independent risk factor for ASCVD, increasing risk two- to threefold in men and even more in women. Women with diabetes are at equivalent CHD risk to men with diabetes. They lose the normally assumed "protection" of the female gender, and their cardiovascular disease rates parallel those of men with diabetes, even before menopause.

The prevalence of lipid abnormalities varies significantly, depending on the characteristics of the study population such as age, gender, type of diabetes, severity of obesity, glycemic control, nondiabetes drugs, and thyroid and renal status. In patients with type 1 diabetes and good glycemic control, lipid levels are no different from an age- and sex-matched control population. In fact, with excellent glycemic control, the lipid profile may show lower total cholesterol and higher HDL cholesterol levels than in control subjects. Levels of cholesterol, ratios of total cholesterol to HDL cholesterol, and triglyceride levels are generally higher in patients with type 1 diabetes during periods of poor glycemic control and then become powerful risk factors for cardiovascular disease. Diabetic ketoacidosis may be associated with a profound temporary hypertriglyceridemia. Although improved glycemic control corrects elevated triglyceride levels and may help to raise HDL cholesterol slightly, a lower A1C will usually not improve LDL cholesterol levels. Separate treatment for LDL cholesterol will be required.

Even minimal microalbuminuria becomes a potent risk factor for CHD and stroke events. When proteinuria reaches the level of early diabetic nephropathy (300–1,000 mg/24 h), the lipid levels may begin to reveal a more atherogenic pattern: falling HDL cholesterol, increased triglyceride levels, and a shift toward larger numbers of smaller, more dense LDL particles without necessarily raising LDL cholesterol levels. The most extreme example is with the nephrotic syndrome. Even when the lipid levels are acceptable by standard lipid profile measures, glycation of lipoproteins and other lipoprotein compositional abnormalities, including oxidation of the LDL particles induced by diabetes and/or hyperglycemia, may make those lipid levels more atherogenic. The precise role of advanced lipid testing for patients with diabetes remains under investigation. Currently, it appears rational to test patients who had reached NCEP ATP III goals but were still believed to be at increased risk or those who had failed to respond clinically to treatment based on standard lipid testing.

Hypertension and cigarette smoking are major cardiovascular risk factors. In health surveys of people age 20–44 yr, 29% of those with diabetes (compared with only 8% of those without diabetes) report having hypertension. Fortunately, the percentage of smokers is decreasing, but young patients with diabetes should always be reminded not to begin this habit and reminded of effects of tobacco on the many complications of diabetes.

In the DCCT, subjects with intensively treated type 1 diabetes and lower A1C levels had trends toward lower levels of LDL cholesterol and fewer myocardial infarctions and peripheral vascular events. Long-term follow-up of the intensively treated group revealed a significant reduction in macrovascular events in this group. Careful analysis of the United Kingdom Prospective Diabetes Study of subjects with type 2 diabetes suggests a role for glycemic control in preventing ASCVD events, particularly when patients achieve an A1C <6.5%. This benefit appears to be independent of the effects of better glycemic control on other cardiovascular risk factors.

ASSESSMENT AND TREATMENT

Because of the high prevalence of cardiovascular risk factors in patients with diabetes and the effect of hyperglycemia to magnify the impact of these risk factors, physicians should consider all patients with type 1 diabetes to be at risk for developing macrovascular disease. They should systematically assess patients for risk factors for ASCVD (those mentioned above plus a family history of cardiovascular disease or hyperlipidemia), question them about symptoms of ASCVD, and be alert for signs of atherosclerosis. When additional risk factors are present, and duration of diabetes enters the late second or third decade, stress testing of asymptomatic patients is appropriate, particularly before a substantial increase in routine physical activity or major surgery. When appropriate, a program for modifying specific risk factors should be started. All patients with type 1 diabetes need to have the critical importance of following a healthy lifestyle reinforced from adolescence, or earlier, into late adult life.

Dyslipidemia

Dyslipidemia in a patient with diabetes may result from poor metabolic control; use of certain drugs, including high-dose β-blockers (other than carvedilol), high-dose diuretics, systemic corticosteroids or other immunosuppressants, protease inhibitor antiviral agents, androgens, progestins (other than micronized progesterone or despironone), or estrogens; obesity; associated conditions such as hypothyroidism, the frequency of which is increased in type 1 diabetes; or an inherited tendency for dyslipidemia. Each cause must be considered in assessing patients with diabetes and abnormal blood lipid levels.

Each year, the American Diabetes Association publishes a revised position statement on the detection and management of lipid disorders in diabetes. It is recommended that adult patients with diabetes undergo annual testing for lipid disorders with fasting serum cholesterol, triglyceride, and HDL cholesterol determinations. If not at goal, more frequent testing may be needed. In adults with low-risk lipid values (LDL <100 mg/dl, HDL >60 mg/dl, triglycerides <150 mg/dl), repeat lipid assessments should be done every 2 yr. In children >2 yr of age, lipid assessment should be done after the diagnosis of diabetes once glucose control has been established. If values are of low risk and there is no family history of dyslipidemia, assessments should be repeated every 5 yr until age 21, then every 2 yr. If abnormalities are identified, more frequent testing is warranted. Children with a family history of dyslipidemia should be assessed annually.

If dyslipidemia is present, the patient should be assessed for factors that aggravate dyslipidemia. Insulin treatment should be intensified in poorly controlled patients, but retesting will be necessary to be sure that additional therapy will be provided if abnormalities persist. Any drugs that might exacerbate hyperlipidemia should be discontinued or reduced where possible. The patient should be evaluated for renal disease and alcohol abuse. Genetic hyperlipidemia, separate from the diabetes, is often the cause of moderate to marked hypercholesterolemia, and the treatment should be based on the etiology of the disorder and not limited to intensified insulin therapy.

The physician should also determine whether the patient is following the current American Diabetes Association guidelines regarding fat intake (see Nutrition, Table 3.9, page 88). Risk categories and recommendations for treatment can be found in Table 6.9. Optimal LDL cholesterol levels for adults with diabetes are <100 mg/dl (<2.60 mmol/l), acceptable HDL cholesterol levels are >40 mg/dl (>1.00 mmol/l) for men and >50 mg/dl (>1.30 mmol/l) for women, and desirable triglyceride levels are <150 mg/dl (<1.68 mmol/l). Patients with diabetes with values other than these should institute medical nutrition therapy (MNT) and

Table 6.9 Category of Risk Based on Lipoprotein Levels for Adults

Risk for Adult Patients with Diabetes	LDL Cholesterol (mg/dl)	HDL Cholesterol (mg/dl)	Triglycerides (mg/dl)
Higher	≥130	<40	≥400
Elevated	100–129	40–59	150–399
Optimal	<100	≥60	<150

From American Diabetes Association Position Statement: see Bibliography, page 226.

exercise. Regarding pharmacological therapy, it is suggested that subjects with type 1 diabetes with clinical CHD and an LDL cholesterol level >100 mg/dl (>2.60 mmol/l) after MNT, exercise, and glucose interventions be treated. For patients with diabetes without preexisting CHD or peripheral arterial or cardiovascular disease, the American Diabetes Association recommendations for starting pharmacological therapy are an LDL cholesterol level ≥130 mg/dl (≥3.35 mmol/l) with a goal of <100 mg/dl (<2.60 mmol/l). However, the recently published Heart Protection Study suggests that there may be benefit in reducing LDL cholesterol by 35–40 mg/dl, even when starting at levels <130 mg/dl. The study included older patients (age 40–80 yr) with type 1 or type 2 diabetes, without apparent difference in benefit based on diabetes type. Although the Veterans Administration HDL Intervention Trial demonstrated a measurable benefit of fibric acid therapy provided to men with low HDL cholesterol (<40 mg/dl [<1.00 mmol/l]) and normal LDL cholesterol (~110 mg/dl [2.85 mmol/l]), this approach has not been evaluated in patients with type 1 diabetes.

Hypertension

Blood pressure should be measured in all patients with type 1 diabetes, including children and adolescents, at each physical examination or at least every 6 mo. Hypertension treatment should be initiated to reduce the risk of macrovascular and microvascular disease. To the extent possible, blood pressure should be maintained at levels <130/80 mmHg in adults or below the 90th percentile for age- and sex-adjusted norms. When prescribing pharmacologic therapy, the clinician should consider the adverse effects of various antihypertensive drugs on hyperglycemia and hypoglycemia, electrolyte balance, renal function, lipid metabolism, ASCVD, and neuropathic symptoms including orthostatic hypotension and impotence (Table 6.10).

Cigarette Smoking

Each patient's smoking history should also be determined. Nonsmokers, particularly children and adolescents, should be encouraged not to begin, and smokers should be strongly urged to stop. The physician's advice not to smoke has an impact and represents time well spent. Advice should be reinforced with educational materials, medications, and referral to a smoking-cessation program.

Table 6.10 Potential Interactions of Antihypertensive Medications in Type 1 Diabetes

Medication	Impact on Glycemia	Advantages	Disadvantages
Diuretics	none (unlike type 2 diabetes, where hypo-kalemia reduces β-cell function)		
Calcium channel blockers	none		edema, increased GI symptoms in patients with neuropathy
Beta-blockers	decreased hypoglycemic awareness		
Angiotensin-converting enzyme (ACE) inhibitors	none	proven to reduce risk of nephropathy	
Angiotensin-receptor blockers (ARBs)	none		
Alpha-blockers	none		increased risk of orthostasis in patients with neuropathy

Advantages and disadvantages are meant to be specific to type 1 diabetes and not to focus on generally appreciated attributes of the drugs.

SYMPTOMS AND SIGNS OF ATHEROSCLEROSIS

The physician should be particularly alert to the symptoms and signs of atherosclerosis in all patients with diabetes.

Cerebrovascular Disease

Symptoms of cerebrovascular disease include intermittent dizziness, transient loss of vision, slurring of speech, and paresthesia or weakness of one arm or leg. Vascular bruits may be heard over the carotid arteries. Noninvasive procedures, including Doppler and carotid ultrasound studies, may be helpful to confirm the diagnosis or detect earlier disease that can still be associated with symptoms.

Aspirin at a dose of 325 mg/day may prevent a recurrence of symptoms, and use of anticoagulant medications after a transient ischemic attack may help some patients. For many patients, 81 mg aspirin/day appears to provide comparable benefit with reduced risk of bleeding. Clopidogrel may be considered in aspirin-intolerant patients or patients who fail to respond to aspirin. Use of aspirin has not been studied in people with diabetes under age 30 yr.

Coronary Heart Disease

As in people without diabetes, CHD may be associated with chest pain or congestive heart failure. However, among people with diabetes, ischemia may occur in the absence of chest pain and particularly in the presence of cardiac autonomic neuropathy. Unexplained onset of congestive heart failure and deterioration of glycemic control to the point of diabetic ketoacidosis may indicate silent myocardial ischemia. Myocardial infarction should be considered in the differential diagnosis of these conditions. Noninvasive procedures, including exercise tolerance tests, exercise thallium studies, and gated blood pool scans, may help establish the diagnosis of silent ischemia and/or myocardial perfusion defects. The utility, frequency, and cost-benefit ratios of these studies in older asymptomatic patients to screen for CHD have not been determined. However, a plan to substantially increase physical activity in a previously inactive patient with long-standing type 1 diabetes should include consideration of stress test evaluation.

Therapy may be medical or surgical. Medical treatments include aspirin, nitrates, calcium-channel blockers, and cardioselective β-adrenergic blockers and agents that modify the renin-angiotensin system. Coronary angiography is necessary if bypass surgery or angioplasty is being considered. Bypass surgery is recommended for left main coronary artery disease and is generally indicated for triple-vessel disease, particularly in the presence of left ventricular dysfunction.

Peripheral Arterial Disease

Peripheral arterial disease should be suspected in patients who complain of buttock, calf, or thigh pain that occurs during exercise and is relieved with rest (intermittent claudication) and/or who exhibit decreased pulses in the lower extremities. The diagnosis can be confirmed with noninvasive Doppler studies. Simple office screens for an abnormal ankle-brachial index (<0.9) can help to detect early disease.

An expert panel of the American Heart Association has recommended regular determination of ankle-brachial index in patients with type 1 diabetes over age 35. Sclerotic vessels can lead to falsely elevated systolic blood pressure and invalid results. Otherwise, a decreased index not only indicates a patient with peripheral arterial disease but is also a strong indicator of possible coronary artery disease and future cardiac mortality.

Treatment with either cilostazol or pentoxifylline may improve symptoms. Aspirin and exercise are important adjuvants to treatment. If pain is incapacitating or persists at rest, or if a foot infection results from impaired blood flow through the major leg arteries, angioplasty or surgery to bypass the diseased vessels may be indicated. Smoking cessation is particularly critical for reduction of symptoms and limb loss.

Aspirin Therapy in Type 1 Diabetes

Aspirin therapy (81–325 mg/day) should be considered as primary prevention in all people with diabetes older than age 30. Use of aspirin has not been studied in individuals with diabetes under the age of 30. Aspirin therapy should be considered in diabetes patients age 21–30 yr if they have any cardiovascular risk factors, e.g., family history of ASCVD, cigarette smoking, hypertension, obesity, micro- or macroalbuminuria, or hyperlipidemia. Aspirin therapy is not recommended for individuals younger than age 21 yr due to the increased risk of Reye's syndrome, which has been associated with aspirin use in this population. People with aspirin allergy, bleeding tendency, anticoagulant therapy, and clinically active hepatic disease are not candidates for aspirin therapy.

CONCLUSION

Patients with type 1 diabetes should be aware of their increased risk of ASCVD and advised of the importance of modifying risk factors such as hypertension, hyperlipidemia, and cigarette smoking. Clinicians should systematically assess patients for risk factors for ASCVD and attempt to modify them. They should question patients about symptoms of ASCVD, examine them for signs of ASCVD, and seek the expertise of appropriate specialists when needed.

BIBLIOGRAPHY

American Diabetes Association: Aspirin therapy in diabetes (Position Statement). *Diabetes Care* 26 (Suppl. 1):S87–S88, 2003

American Diabetes Association: Management of dyslipidemia in adults with diabetes (Position Statement). *Diabetes Care* 26 (Suppl. 1):S83–S86, 2003

American Diabetes Association: Smoking and diabetes (Position Statement). *Diabetes Care* 26 (Suppl. 1):S89–S90, 2003

American Diabetes Association: Treatment of hypertension in adults with diabetes (Position Statement). *Diabetes Care* 26 (Suppl. 1):S80–S82, 2003

Campos H, Moye LA, Glasser SP, Stampfer MJ, Sacks FM: Low-density lipoprotein size, pravastatin treatment, and coronary events. *JAMA* 286:1468–1474, 2001

DCCT Research Group: The effect of intensive treatment of diabetes on the development and progression of long-term complications on insulin-dependent diabetes mellitus. *N Engl J Med* 329:977–986, 1993

Fielding JE: Smoking: health effects and control. *N Engl J Med* 313:491–498, 555–560, 1985

Garg A: Management of dyslipidemia in IDDM patients. *Diabetes Care* 17:224–234, 1994

Grundy SM, Balady GJ, Criqui MH, Fletcher G, Greenland P, Hiratzka LF, Houston-Miller N, Kris-Etherton P, Krumholz HM, LaRosa J, Ockene IS, Pearson TA, Reed J, Smith SC, Washington R: When to start cholesterol-lowering therapy in patients with coronary heart disease: statement for health care professionals from the American Heart Association Task Force on Risk Reduction. *Circulation* 95:1683–1685, 1997

Heart Protection Study Collaborative Group: MRC/BHF Heart Protection Study of cholesterol lowering with simvastatin in 20536 high-risk individuals: a randomised placebo-controlled study. *Lancet* 360:7–22, 2002

Kannel WB, McGee DL: Diabetes and glucose tolerance as risk factors for cardiovascular disease: the Framingham study. *Diabetes Care* 2:120–126, 1979

Lipid Research Clinics Program: The Lipid Research Clinics coronary primary prevention trial results. *JAMA* 251:351–374, 1984

Robins SJ, Collins D, Wittes JT, Papademetriou V, Deedwania PC, Schaefer EJ, McNamara JR, Kashyap ML, Hershman JM, Wexler LF, Rubins HB, VA-HIT Study Group: Relation of gemfibrozil treatment and lipids levels with major coronary events: VA-HIT: a randomized controlled trial. *JAMA* 285:1585–1591, 2001

Suarez L, Barrett-Connor E: Interaction between cigarette smoking and diabetes mellitus in the prediction of death attributed to cardiovascular disease. *Am J Epidemiol* 120:670–675, 1984

Turner RC, Millns H, Neil HA, Stratton IM, Manley SE, Mathews DR, Holman DR: Risk factor for coronary artery disease in non-insulin dependent diabetes mellitus (UKPDS 23). *Br Med J* 316:823–828, 1998

LIMITED JOINT MOBILITY

Limited joint mobility (LJM) is a potentially important clinical marker for diabetes complications such as retinopathy, nephropathy, neuropathy, statural growth abnormalities, hypertension, and hepatomegaly. Glycation of tissue proteins associated with chronic hyperglycemia may be responsible for many long-term complications, including LJM.

DETECTION AND EVALUATION

LJM may occur in children or adults, is painless, and causes little disability. Thus, it is unlikely to be brought to the attention of family members or health professionals. The only way to detect LJM is to examine hands and joints as part of routine physical examinations.

To evaluate for LJM, the following should be included. Observe and shake both hands of the patient, noting any scleroderma-like stiffness of the skin. The patient should then be asked to place the hands in a clapping or "prayer" position with forearms as parallel to the floor as possible (Fig. 6.10). Any inability to oppose the joints of the fingers and any limitation of flexion or extension of wrist, elbow, neck, or spine should be documented.

If pain or neuromuscular findings (e.g., atrophy, paresthesia) are present, other disorders, such as tenosynovitis or carpal tunnel syndrome, should be con-

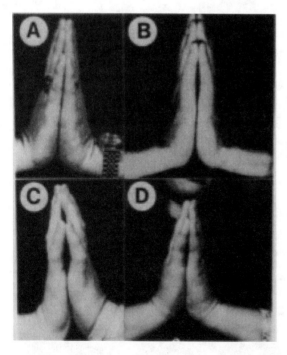

Figure 6.10 Limited joint mobility of increasing severity. *A*: normal joint mobility. *B*: bilateral contracture of 5th fingers. *C*: bilateral contracture of more than 5th fingers. *D*: bilateral wrist involvement.

sidered. In adults, another possibility is Dupuytren's contracture, which is painless and characterized by palmar nodules and involvement of the third and fourth fingers.

Because there is a relationship between the severity of LJM and the microvascular complications of diabetes, patients found to have LJM at an office visit should be carefully examined for clinical evidence of retinopathy via ophthalmoscopy; for nephropathy by a quantitative determination of urinary microalbumin excretion; and for hypertension, hepatomegaly, and neuropathy by careful clinical examination.

CONCLUSION

Until intervention in the primary glycation process becomes possible or better treatment strategies are perfected, patients with LJM should be periodically assessed for complications and should strive for the best possible glycemic control.

BIBLIOGRAPHY

Aljahlan M, Lee KC, Toth E: Limited joint mobility in diabetes. *Postgrad Med* 105:99–101, 105–106, 1999

Brink SJ: *Pediatric and Adolescent Diabetes Mellitus.* Chicago, IL, Year Book, 1987

Duffin AC, Conaghue KC, Potter M, McInnes A, Chan AK, King J, Howard NJ, Silink M: Limited joint mobility in the hands and feet of adolescents with type 1 diabetes mellitus. *Diabet Med* 16:125–30, 1999

Frost D, Beischer W: Limited joint mobility in type 1 diabetic patients: associations with microangiopathy and subclinical macroangiopathy are different in men and women. *Diabetes Care* 24:95–99, 2001

Rosenbloom AL: Skeletal and joint manifestations of childhood diabetes. *Pediatr Clin N Am* 31:569–590, 1984

GROWTH

Abnormalities of height (absolute short stature as well as decreased growth velocity) are known consequences of insulin deficiency. Although the classic example occurs in the extreme and relatively rare Mauriac syndrome (diabetic dwarfism), subtle abnormalities of growth and development are not uncommon among youngsters with type 1 diabetes. Patients with poorly controlled diabetes have decreased insulin-like growth factor-1 levels and paradoxical increments in growth hormone levels during the night and in response to provocative stimuli. These abnormalities can be prevented or corrected with better glycemic control.

MAURIAC SYNDROME

Children with Mauriac syndrome are markedly delayed in linear growth and sexual maturation. They are usually pale, appear chronically ill, and have generalized puffiness of the face and extremities and a protuberant abdomen. LJM and hepatomegaly are often present, and laboratory analysis includes not only hyperglycemia and elevated A1C levels but also hyperlipidemia.

SUBTLE GROWTH ABNORMALITIES

Less marked growth abnormalities become apparent when large patient populations are studied and subtle growth changes are sought, including a lag in height or weight or a deviation from previously established growth curves (Figs. 6.11 and 6.12). Defined in this fashion, 5–10% of youngsters with type 1 diabetes will not

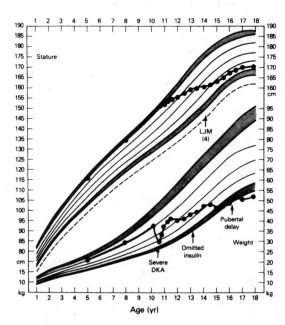

Figure 6.11 Inadequate diabetes control and growth abnormalities. Growth deceleration solely from uncontrolled diabetes mellitus. Patient refused to take 2 shots of insulin each day. Most of the time, patient omitted morning insulin and refused to follow any type of meal plan. The family refused psychiatric consultation. Adapted from Brink SJ: see Bibliography, page 232.

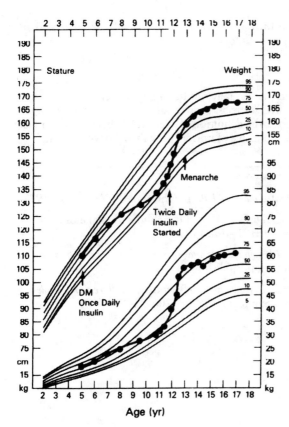

Figure 6.12 Catch-up growth phenomenon with adequate insulin. Growth data from child with type 1 diabetes treated with 1 shot of morning insulin, showing growth deceleration and catch-up growth phenomenon after twice-daily insulin was started. Adapted from Brink SJ: see Bibliography, page 232.

grow well. Children most likely to be affected are those with the earliest onset of diabetes and those who have the worst day-to-day glycemic control and the highest A1C levels. Boys are two or three times more likely to have a growth abnormality than girls.

DETERMINING GROWTH RATE

The only way to determine whether growth is adequate is to measure height and weight at each office visit and to plot data on standardized growth charts. Ideally, data should be recorded at least every 3–4 mo; at minimum, height and weight should be measured and recorded annually. Growth data obtained from other family members may be extremely valuable in placing an individual youngster's growth in perspective. Bone age determination (single radiograph of left wrist and hand compared with standard radiographs) coupled with other hormonal measurements may help assess the need for further evaluation. If growth abnormalities are found, metabolic status should be carefully evaluated and appropriate recommendation for improvement made, such as changing to an intensified insulin treatment program.

CONCLUSION

Although mild growth retardation may not be totally preventable, evidence strongly indicates that major alterations in growth rate can be avoided by better blood glucose control. Therefore, the definition of adequate diabetes control must include the attainment and maintenance of normal growth and development.

BIBLIOGRAPHY

Brink SJ: *Pediatric and Adolescent Diabetes Mellitus.* Chicago, IL, Year Book, 1987

Clarke WL, Vance ML, Rogol AD: Growth and the child with diabetes mellitus. *Diabetes Care* 16 (Suppl. 3):101–106, 1993

Jackson RL, Guthrie RA: *The Physiological Management of Diabetes in Children.* New York, Medical Examination Publishing, 1986

Travis LB, Brouhard BJ, Schreiner BK: *Diabetes Mellitus in Children and Adolescence.* Philadelphia, PA, WB Saunders, 1987, p. 206–210

Emerging Therapies

Highlights

New Insulin Analogs
Insulin Detemir
Insulin Glulisine

Alternative Insulin Delivery Systems
Pulmonary Insulin
Peritoneal Insulin

Other Islet Cell Hormones
Amylin Analog Pramlintide
Islet Neogenesis–Associated Protein (INGAP)

Islet Transplantation

Highlights
Emerging Therapies

NEW INSULIN ANALOGS

■ Insulin detemir represents a new class of soluble analogs of human insulin with a prolonged duration of action that provides effective glycemic control in type 1 and type 2 diabetes. Insulin detemir has demonstrated less nocturnal hypoglycemia, lower fasting blood glucose, less within-patient variability, and less weight gain than human NPH insulin and a comparable safety profile.

■ Insulin glulisine is a new rapid-acting insulin analog that has shown a time-action profile similar to other rapid-acting analogs with no safety issues in phase I studies.

ALTERNATIVE INSULIN DELIVERY SYSTEMS

■ Studies have shown that inhaled insulin is absorbed more rapidly than subcutaneous regular insulin and as quickly as rapid-acting insulin in patients with type 1 and type 2 diabetes. Approximately 10–30% of inhaled insulin is absorbed into the circulation. Results from ongoing clinical trials have shown that the inhaled insulin preparations being studied are as effective as subcutaneous insulin preparations in type 1 and type 2 diabetes, with hypoglycemia the most frequently reported adverse event.

■ Clinical studies have shown that peritoneal insulin delivery via implantable insulin pumps is a safe and effective mechanism for achieving good glycemic control with a low rate of severe hypoglycemia. Candidates for implantable insulin pumps include patients having difficulty maintaining consistent glycemic control, those with frequent severe hypoglycemia episodes, patients with subcutaneous insulin absorption resistance and injection or infusion skin reactions, and those who have not responded well to intensive insulin therapy.

OTHER ISLET CELL HORMONES

■ Pramlintide is a soluble nonaggregating amylin analog in development as a possible adjunct to insulin therapy. The clinical benefits of pramlintide are achieved by replacing the action of amylin, a naturally occurring β-cell hormone that is deficient in type 1 diabetes. Results from clinical studies showed that when pramlintide was added to insulin regimens, patients with type 1 diabetes had improved glycemic control with no increased body weight or severe hypoglycemia.

■ Islet neogenesis–associated protein (INGAP) is a peptide capable of stimulating islet cell neogenesis and lowering blood glucose levels. Studies in several animal models of type 1 diabetes showed that the INGAP peptide reversed diabetes by stimulating new islet cell growth. Clinical trials are ongoing in type 1 diabetes.

ISLET TRANSPLANTATION

■ Significant progress has been made in human islet allotransplantation over the past several years, and most patients have achieved insulin independence, with normalization of A1C at 1 yr post–islet transplantation. These results have not occurred without complications, the most significant of which is hepatic bleeding due to the administration of islets into the portal vein in 7% of patients. As a result of this and other potential risks from immunotherapy, most islet transplants to date have been done in patients with recurrent, refractory, severe hypoglycemia or marked glycemic instability. However, research is ongoing to improve these results, minimizing the risks from immunotherapy and developing other potential sources of islet cells.

Emerging Therapies

There are many new treatment strategies in development for type 1 diabetes. This chapter will discuss treatments and drugs that are in the final stages of development (phase II or III trials) and most likely will gain FDA approval in the next few years.

NEW INSULIN ANALOGS

INSULIN DETEMIR

The long-acting analog insulin detemir represents a new class of soluble analogs of human insulin intended to cover basal insulin requirements. Compared to the structure of human insulin, the amino acid residue in position B30 of insulin detemir has been omitted, and a 14-carbon fatty acid chain has been attached to position B29. The fatty acid chain attached to position B29 binds to the fatty acid binding sites of albumin in the subcutaneous tissue, delaying absorption to the bloodstream. Approximately 98–99% of insulin detemir is bound to albumin in plasma. The prolonged duration of action is attributable to increased self-association at the injection site and albumin binding. The rate of absorption is limited by the low concentration of free insulin detemir available for diffusion through tissues and passage across the capillary wall.

Based on phase III trials, insulin detemir shows all the desired properties of a basal insulin. In the eight trials with insulin-treated subjects with type 1 or type 2 diabetes, the use of insulin detemir resulted in glycemic control similar to that attained with NPH insulin (noninferiority was confirmed). In subjects with type 1 diabetes, the self-measured blood glucose profiles at the end of the treatment periods appeared in general to be flatter with insulin detemir treatment than with NPH, reflecting more stable glucose levels during the day and especially during the night. This is in accord with the reduction in the risk of nocturnal hypoglycemic episodes found with insulin detemir compared to NPH in subjects with type 1 diabetes. Studies comparing the effectiveness of insulin detemir to insulin glargine have not been done as of early 2003.

There is no evidence suggesting any kind of safety risk of insulin detemir other than that normally associated with the taking of insulin. The risk of hypoglycemia, particularly nocturnal hypoglycemia, was consistently lower with insulin detemir versus NPH, although the risk of major hypoglycemic episodes was similar. One clear benefit that emerged unexpectedly from the clinical development program was the weight neutrality of insulin detemir. Although subjects on NPH gained weight in every trial, subjects taking insulin detemir maintained their weight or had slight reductions.

In conclusion, insulin detemir offers effective glycemic control with lower within-subject variability and less weight gain and a similar safety profile compared to human NPH insulin. Insulin detemir can be administered once or twice daily, thus allowing the treatment regimen to be tailored to individual subject needs. Insulin detemir was filed with the FDA in December 2002.

INSULIN GLULISINE

Insulin glulisine (3^BLys-29^B-Glu-human insulin) is a new rapid-acting insulin analog under development. As with other rapid-acting analogs, substitution of certain amino acids has created a tendency of the insulin molecule to disperse from hexamers into monomers very quickly on injection. Phase I studies have shown a time-action profile similar to other rapid-acting analogs with no safety issues observed. Preclinical toxicology studies have not demonstrated any untoward toxicity. Phase III trials are under clinical development as of December 2002.

BIBLIOGRAPHY

Frick A, Becker R, Wessels D, Scholtz H: Pharmacokinetic and glucodynamic profiles of insulin glulisine following subcutaneous administration at various injection sites (Abstract). *Diabetes* 52 (Suppl. 1): A119, 2003

Kurtzhals P, Havelund S, Jonassen I, Kiehr B, Larsen UD, Ribel U, Markussen J: Albumin-binding of insulins acylated with fatty-acids: characterization of the ligand protein-interaction and correlation between binding-affinity and timing of the insulin effect *in-vivo*. *Biochem J* 312:725–731, 1995

Standl E, Roberts A, Draeger E: Long-term efficacy and safety of insulin detemir in subjects with type 1 diabetes: favorable weight development and risk reduction of nocturnal hypoglycemia (Abstract). *Diabetes* 51 (Suppl. 2):A115, 2002

Vague P, Selam J-L, Skeie S, de Leeuw I, Elte JWF, Haahr H, Kristensen A, Draeger E: Insulin detemir is associated with more predictable glycemic control and reduced risk of hypoglycemia than NPH insulin in patients with type 1 diabetes on a basal-bolus regimen with premeal insulin aspart. *Diabetes Care* 26:590–596, 2003

Werner U, Gerlach M, Hofmann M, Seipke G: Insulin glulisine is a novel, parenteral human insulin analog with a rapid-acting time-action profile: a crossover, euglycemic clamp study in normoglycemic dogs (Abstract). *Diabetes* 52 (Suppl. 1): A138, 2003

ALTERNATIVE INSULIN DELIVERY SYSTEMS

Multiple alternative methods for delivering insulin into the bloodstream are under development and investigation. Two methodologies that are currently in phase III studies are pulmonary insulin delivery via inhalation and peritoneal insulin delivery via implantable pumps and are discussed below. Transdermal and buccal insulin delivery are also under development but are only in phase I and II trials and therefore will not be discussed below.

PULMONARY INSULIN

Pulmonary delivery of insulin in humans was initially reported in 1925, with further studies in the 1970s and 1980s confirming the feasibility of administering insulin by the aerosol route. In these studies, ~10–30% of the insulin inhaled was absorbed into the circulation, and the aerosols appeared to be well tolerated. Since then, all insulin manufacturers in the world have partnered with various pharmaceutical and device companies to clinically develop their own pulmonary insulin systems.

Studies in patients with type 1 or type 2 diabetes have shown that inhaled insulin is absorbed more rapidly than subcutaneous regular insulin and as quickly as rapid-acting insulin (aspart/lispro). Duration of action of inhaled insulin is longer than rapid-acting insulin and similar to regular insulin. The bioavailability of inhaled insulin relative to subcutaneous regular insulin is ~10% with all the current inhaled systems in development except for technosphere insulin, which has ~30% bioavailability. The intrasubject variability of inhaled insulin is comparable to subcutaneous regular insulin. Studies in smokers and chronic obstructive pulmonary disease patients have shown enhanced absorption of inhaled insulin, with studies in asthma patients showing some decreased absorption. Results of studies in patients with rhinovirus infection have been mixed, with most showing no substantial change in the pharmacokinetics of inhaled insulin.

Phase I, II, and III trials are ongoing, with four different preparations of inhaled insulin. Results from these trials to date have shown that inhaled insulin regimens are as effective as subcutaneous insulin regimens in type 1 and type 2 diabetes patients. In type 2 diabetes patients, adding inhaled insulin to oral agent failures showed a marked improvement in glycated hemoglobin (A1C) compared to continuing oral agents alone. Quality of life and treatment satisfaction assessments have shown inhaled insulin therapy is preferred over subcutaneous insulin therapy by many patients.

In all clinical studies, the most frequently reported adverse event is hypoglycemia. Mild changes in pulmonary function have been reported with a 1–5% decline in forced expiratory volume at 1 s (FEV1) and in carbon monoxide diffusion capacity (DL_{co}). A ≥15% decline in FEV1 and DL_{co} occurred in a small subset of patients. The importance of these changes as well as any long-term clinical sequelae are unknown. As a result, long-term trials are ongoing to answer these questions.

PERITONEAL INSULIN

Continuous peritoneal insulin infusions via programmable implantable insulin pumps have been used for the last 20 yr. Original manufacturers included Infusaid, Medtronic MiniMed, and Siemens Promedos, although only Medtronic MiniMed is currently known to be pursuing implantable pump research and manufacturing.

The Medtronic MiniMed 2007 pump, which measures 3.2 inches in diameter and 0.8 inches in thickness, has a weight of 4.6 oz before filling and a reservoir volume of 15 ml. Safety features of the pump include a positive displacement piston design and a negative pressure reservoir for filling. A specially formulated U-400 type of insulin has been developed to last for 2–3 mo between refills. Refills are accomplished by inserting a needle through the skin into the pump. An external electronic communicator allows the patient to control pump operation similar to the manner an external insulin pump is programmed. A side port allows direct access to the delivery cannula for clearing occlusions. About 1,000 people with diabetes have received an implanted insulin pump as of December 2002. The pump is approved for commercial sale in Europe, with both the insulin and pump awaiting approval by the FDA in the US.

Intraperitoneal insulin is rapidly and predictably absorbed into the portal circulation simulating physiologic insulin delivery and absorption. Such rapid and predictable absorption may avoid the peripheral hyperinsulinemia seen with most insulin regimens and the theoretical risk of accelerated atherosclerosis. Clinical studies have proven implantable pump therapy to be safe and effective for achieving glycemic control (significant reductions in A1C, average glucose level, and glucose variability), decreasing the rate of severe hypoglycemia, and improving glucagon responses to hypoglycemia. One study demonstrated a reduction in hypoglycemic events with an average rate as low as four events per 100 patient-years. Other benefits may include physiological lipid metabolism and improvements in quality of life.

Appropriate candidates include

- diabetes patients who have difficulty maintaining consistent glycemic control
- those with frequent severe hypoglycemic events
- those who have not responded well to intensive insulin therapy
- those with subcutaneous insulin absorption resistance and injection or infusion site skin reactions

Use of a long-term glucose sensor connected to the implantable pump is under clinical investigation. The glucose sensor is inserted into the superior vena cava and measures blood glucose continually via a glucose oxidase electrode. The sensor is powered by the implantable pump and has been shown to produce accurate glucose measurements for >14 mo with weekly calibrations. Pilot studies to close the loop and deliver insulin in response to blood glucose levels have been reported. Efforts are under way with several different methodologies to close the loop using continuous subcutaneous glucose systems connected to external pumps, as well as implanted sensors connected to external or implantable sensors.

BIBLIOGRAPHY

Duckworth WC, Saudek CD, Henry RR: Why intraperitoneal delivery of insulin with implantable pumps in NIDDM? *Diabetes* 41:657–661, 1992

Dunn FL, Nathan DM, Scavini M, Selam JL, Wingrove TG, the Implantable Insulin Pump Trial Study Group: Long-term therapy of IDDM with an implantable insulin pump. *Diabetes Care* 20:59–63, 1997

Hanaire-Broutin H, Broussolie C, Jeandidier N, Renard E, Guerci B, Haardt M-J, Lassmann-Vague V, the EVADIAC Study Group (Evaluation dans le Diabète du Traitement par Implants Actifs): Feasibility of intraperitoneal insulin therapy with programmable implantable pumps in IDDM: a multi-center study. *Diabetes Care* 18:388–392, 1995

Henry RR, Mudaliar SRD, Howland WC III, Chu N, Kim D, An B, Reinhardt RR: Inhaled insulin using the AERx insulin Diabetes Management System in healthy and asthmatic subjects. *Diabetes Care* 26:764–769, 2003

Renard E, Shah R, Miller M, Starkweather T, Kolopp M, Costalat G, Bringer J: Accuracy of real-time blood glucose measurement by long-term sensor system allows automated insulin delivery in diabetic patients (Abstract). *Diabetes* 51 (Suppl. 2):A126, 2002

Saudek CD, Selam JL, Pitt HA, Waxman K, Rubio M, Jeandidier N, Rurner D, Fischell RE, Charles MA: A preliminary trial of the Programmable Implantable Medication System for insulin delivery. *N Engl J Med* 321:574–579, 1989

Skyler JS, Cefalu WT, Kourides IA, Landschulz WH, Balagtas CC, Cheng SL, Gelfard RA: Efficacy of inhaled human insulin in type 1 diabetes mellitus: a randomized proof-of-concept study. *Lancet* 357:331–335, 2001

Steil GM, Blumauer N, Leech J, Long K, Panteleon AE, Rebrin K: Closed loop insulin delivery using subcutaneous (sc) glucose sensing and sc insulin delivery (Abstract). *Diabetes* 50 (Suppl. 2):A132, 2001

OTHER ISLET CELL HORMONES

AMYLIN ANALOG PRAMLINTIDE

Type 1 diabetes manifests with absolute insulin deficiency, and for the past 80 yr, insulin replacement therapy has been the only pharmacological treatment available for this disease. Despite considerable advances in insulin therapy, such as the development of insulin pumps and, more recently, rapid- and long-acting insulin analogs, many patients with type 1 diabetes are still unable to achieve and maintain optimal glycemic control. Among the clinical barriers that hinder the attainment of glycemic goals with insulin therapy alone are the increased risk of hypoglycemia, postprandial hyperglycemia, excessive glucose fluctuations throughout the day, and undesired weight gain (Table 7.1). More recently, it has been recognized that pancreatic β-cells secrete another glucoregulatory hormone, amylin, that is normally cosecreted with insulin in response to meals. Consequently, the autoimmune-mediated destruction of pancreatic β-cells in type 1 diabetes results in an absolute deficiency not only of insulin, but also of amylin.

Amylin is a 37–amino acid neuroendocrine hormone that binds with high affinity to certain areas of the brain and complements the effects of insulin in postprandial glucose control ("partner hormone" of insulin). Specifically, while insulin is the major hormone in the regulation of glucose disposal (efflux) out of the circulation, amylin regulates the inflow of glucose into the circulation after meals. This is achieved by suppression of glucagon secretion and regulation of gastric emptying. In addition, amylin has been shown to reduce food intake and body weight in laboratory animals, suggesting that it may also act as a physiological satiety signal.

The findings that amylin is normally cosecreted with insulin, that it complements the effect of insulin, and that it is completely deficient in type 1 diabetes led

Table 7.1 Pramlintide Effect in Type 1 Diabetes

Unresolved Problems with Insulin Therapy	Pramlintide Effect
Suboptimal glycemic control in many patients	Additional, sustained reduction in A1C (~0.3–0.5%)
Failure to achieve recommended glycemic control (A1C <7%)	Increased proportion of patients achieve A1C <7%
Postprandial hyperglycemia	Marked reduction in postprandial glucose excursions
Excessive diurnal glucose fluctuations	Reduction of glucose fluctuations
Increased risk of severe hypoglycemia	No overall increase in severe hypoglycemic event rate
Excessive weight gain	Weight loss, confined to overweight and obese patients

to the hypothesis that amylin replacement may convey additional benefits to patients with type 1 diabetes when added to existing insulin regimens. Human amylin itself is not optimal for clinical use because of its insolubility and tendency to self-aggregate; thus, a soluble nonaggregating equipotent amylin analog, pramlintide, was developed.

Pramlintide is in late-stage clinical development as a possible adjunct to insulin therapy in people with type 1 or type 2 diabetes. Like insulin, pramlintide is given via subcutaneous injection.

In short-term studies (days or weeks) of patients with type 1 diabetes, addition of pramlintide to insulin injections before meals reduced postprandial glucose excursions by at least 75%, regardless of whether pramlintide was used with regular insulin or a rapid-acting insulin analog. Adjunctive treatment with pramlintide reduced excessive glucose fluctuations over the course of the day, as demonstrated in a 4-wk study with a continuous glucose-monitoring device in an intensively treated type 1 diabetes patient (Fig. 7.1). Note that these effects were achieved with pramlintide doses (30 and 60 µg) that yield a plasma pramlintide profile similar to the normal postprandial amylin response in healthy subjects, indicating that the improvement in postprandial glucose control is achieved via physiological replacement of the absent amylin action. Additional studies in patients with type 1 diabetes have shown that the improvement in postprandial glucose control with pramlintide is attributable to both a correction of postprandial glucagon hypersecretion, thereby controlling excessive glucose inflow from the liver, and a slowing of gastric emptying, thereby controlling glucose inflow from the gut. These pramlintide effects are entirely consistent with the known physiological functions of amylin.

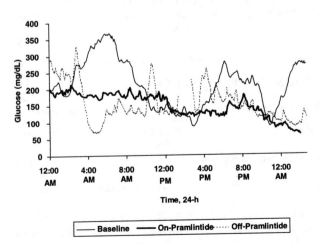

Figure 7.1 Glucose profile over 24 h before, during, and after pramlintide treatment in a type 1 diabetes patient on intensive therapy with an insulin pump.

In long-term studies (6 or 12 mo) in patients with type 1 diabetes, addition of pramlintide to preexisting insulin regimens led to a significant A1C reduction of ~0.3–0.5% compared to placebo and a doubling of the proportion of patients achieving recommended glycemic targets (A1C <7%). This makes pramlintide the first pharmacological agent and hormone replacement other than insulin shown to improve long-term glycemic control in patients with type 1 diabetes. It is important to note that the glycemic improvement with pramlintide was not accompanied by the long-term increases in body weight and severe hypoglycemia typically seen when glycemic control is improved by increasing the dose of insulin. On the contrary, compared to placebo, pramlintide treatment was associated with a relative decrease in insulin use and reduction in body weight that was most pronounced (~1.5–3 kg) in overweight and obese patients (lean patients did not have unwarranted weight loss). Pramlintide treatment was generally well tolerated; the most common adverse event was mild nausea, which typically occurred during the first few weeks of therapy and dissipated over time.

In summary, amylin replacement with pramlintide elicits a combination of clinical benefits that addresses some of the unresolved challenges with insulin therapy in type 1 diabetes (Table 7.1). Adjunctive therapy with pramlintide might therefore hold particular promise for those patients with type 1 diabetes in whom excessive unpredictable glucose fluctuations, postprandial hyperglycemia, undesired weight gain, or repeated episodes of insulin-induced hypoglycemia hinder the achievement of glycemic targets. The clinical benefits of pramlintide are achieved by replacing the action of a second, naturally occurring β-cell hormone that is deficient in type 1 diabetes. By better matching the rate of glucose inflow to the rate of insulin-mediated glucose disposal, pramlintide improves glucose control via a unique mechanism of action that is distinct from, and complementary to, the action of insulin and its analogs. If approved, pramlintide may become the first novel therapy for type 1 diabetes in 80 yr that, when used with insulin, may assist patients with type 1 diabetes in the pursuit of optimal glycemic control.

Table 7.1 Pramlintide Effect in Type 1 Diabetes

Unresolved Problems with Insulin Therapy	Pramlintide Effect
Suboptimal glycemic control in many patients	Additional, sustained reduction in A1C (~0.3–0.5%)
Failure to achieve recommended glycemic control (A1C <7%)	Increased proportion of patients achieve A1C <7%
Postprandial hyperglycemia	Marked reduction in postprandial glucose excursions
Excessive diurnal glucose fluctuations	Reduction of glucose fluctuations
Increased risk of severe hypoglycemia	No overall increase in severe hypoglycemic event rate
Excessive weight gain	Weight loss, confined to overweight and obese patients

ISLET NEOGENESIS–ASSOCIATED PROTEIN

Islet neogenesis–associated protein (INGAP) is a peptide that is capable of stimulating islet cell neogenesis and lowering blood glucose levels. It was discovered in the 1990s and is currently made by recombinant techniques. A 15– amino acid segment has been isolated as the active peptide of the INGAP protein. In several animal models of type 1 diabetes, the INGAP peptide has been shown to reverse diabetes by stimulation of new islet cell growth. Early phase I trials in humans have shown no adverse effect of the peptide in healthy volunteers. Phase II trials are underway to see whether the INGAP peptide has similar effects in humans with type 1 diabetes. If successful and without any major adverse events, this peptide could dramatically change the future treatment of both type 1 and type 2 diabetes.

BIBLIOGRAPHY

Baron AD, Kim D, Weyer C: Novel peptides under development for the treatment of type 1 and type 2 diabetes. *Curr Drug Targets Immune Endocr Metabol Disord* 2:63–82, 2002

Buse JB, Weyer C, Maggs DG: Amylin replacement with pramlintide in type 1 and type 2 diabetes: a physiological approach to overcome barriers with insulin therapy. *Clinical Diabetes* 20:137–144, 2002

Edelman SV, Weyer C: Unresolved challenges with insulin therapy in type 1 and type 2 diabetes: potential benefit of replacing amylin, a second β-cell hormone. *Diabetes Technol Ther* 4:175–189, 2002

Gottlieb A, Velte M, Fineman M, Kolterman O: Pramlintide as an adjunct to insulin therapy improved glycemic and weight control in people with type 1 diabetes during treatment for 52 weeks (Abstract). *Diabetes* 49 (Suppl. 1):A109, 2000

Levetan C, Want LL, Weyer C, Strobel SA, Crean J, Wang Y, Maggs DG, Kolterman OG, Chandran M, Mudaliar SR, Henry RR: Impact of pramlintide on glucose fluctuations and postprandial glucose, glucagon, and triglyceride excursions among patients with type 1 diabetes intensively treated with insulin pumps. *Diabetes Care* 26:1–8, 2003

Nyholm B, Brock B, Ørskov L, Schmitz O: Amylin receptor agonists: a novel pharmacological approach in the management of insulin-treated diabetes mellitus. *Expert Opin Investig Drugs* 10:1–12, 2001

Weyer C, Maggs DG, Kim D, Crean J, Wang Y, Burrell T, Fineman M, Kornstein J, Schwartz S, Guiterrez M, Kolterman OG: Mealtime amylin replacement with pramlintide markedly improves postprandial glucose excursions when added to regular insulin or insulin lispro in patients with type 1 diabetes: a dose-timing study. *Diabetologia* 45 (Suppl. 2):A240, 2002

Weyer C, Maggs DG, Young AA, Kolterman OG: Amylin replacement with pramlintide as an adjunct to insulin therapy in type 1 and type 2 diabetes mellitus: a physiological approach toward improved metabolic control. *Curr Pharm Des* 7:1353–1373, 2001

Whitehouse F, Kruger DF, Fineman M, Shen L, Ruggles JA, Maggs DG, Weyer C, Kolterman OG: A randomized study and open-label extension evaluating the long-term efficacy of pramlintide as an adjunct to insulin therapy in type 1 diabetes. *Diabetes Care* 25:724–730, 2002

ISLET TRANSPLANTATION

Significant progress in the field of islet transplantation has occurred over the past several years. In July 2000, a team from University of Alberta in Edmonton reported success in achieving up to 14 mo of insulin independence with normalization of A1C and resolution of recurrent severe hypoglycemia in seven type 1 diabetes patients by human islet allotransplantation from cadaver pancreases. Their success has been attributed to improved human islet isolation and purification procedures, along with different immunosuppression regimens that avoid the use of glucocorticoids and cyclosporine, which have in the past been shown toxic to the islets. Since their initial report, hundreds of other islet allotransplantations into the portal vein of the liver have been done around the world in designated research centers using variations of the Edmonton protocol. At one year post–islet transplantation, >80% have achieved insulin independence with normalization of A1C. More than one cadaver pancreas has been used at staged procedures in most patients, with some requiring islets from three or more cadaver pancreases.

Such success in human islet allotransplantation has not occurred without risks and complications to the patients. The most significant complication has been hepatic bleeding in 11%, with two reported cases of portal vein thrombosis. As a result, some centers are using an open laparotomy approach to administer the islets into the portal vein instead of a percutaneous transhepatic approach. Other complications have been minor, with mouth ulcerations from sirolimus in 84%, transient rise in liver enzymes in 56%, the need for statin therapy in 39%, renal dysfunction in 6%, severe neutropenia in 5%, and rare cases of pneumonitis, with one death from pneumonitis reported in a European center. No cancers or infection with cytomegalovirus have been reported as of December 2002.

As a result of these risks, islet allotransplantation is only recommended to patients where the benefits of improved metabolic control with avoidance of severe hypoglycemia are greater than the risks of the islet allotransplantation procedure and the ongoing risks of chronic immunosuppression. Most islet transplants to date have been done in patients with recurrent, refractory, severe hypoglycemia or marked glycemic instability. It is not known yet whether such transplantation will reverse or stop microvascular complications, because glucose intolerance persists.

Additional research is ongoing in multiple areas to improve the current clinical results. These areas involve

- improvement in islet yield from cadaver pancreases
- refinements to the protocol to improve engraftment
- long-term prevention and recurrence of autoimmunity
- development of safe immunomodulation strategies
- achievement of donor-specific immune tolerance

If success is achieved in these areas, the critical challenge will be to identify sufficient and suitable sources of insulin-producing tissue to treat the large number of patients who could benefit from this therapy. For these reasons, research on xenogeneic islets, embryonic and adult stem cells, islet regeneration and proliferation, and engineering of insulin-producing cells must be continued. It is important to identify the ideal source of insulin-producing tissue that will be utilized on a large scale once the current impediments and limitations of immuno-suppression are resolved.

BIBLIOGRAPHY

Shapiro AMJ, Lakey JRT, Ryan EA, Korbutt GS, Toth E, Warnock GL, Kneteman NM, Rajotte RV: Islet transplantation in seven patients with type 1 diabetes using a glucocorticoid-free immunosuppressive regimen. *N Engl J Med* 343:230–238, 2000

Index

About the American Diabetes Association

The American Diabetes Association is the nation's leading voluntary health organization supporting diabetes research, information, and advocacy. Its mission is to prevent and cure diabetes and to improve the lives of all people affected by diabetes. The American Diabetes Association is the leading publisher of comprehensive diabetes information. Its huge library of practical and authoritative books for people with diabetes covers every aspect of self-care—cooking and nutrition, fitness, weight control, medications, complications, emotional issues, and general self-care.

To order American Diabetes Association books: Call 1-800-232-6733. Or log on to http://store.diabetes.org

To join the American Diabetes Association: Call 1-800-806-7801. www.diabetes.org/membership

For more information about diabetes or ADA programs and services: Call 1-800-342-2383. E-mail: Customerservice@diabetes.org or log on to www.diabetes.org

To locate an ADA/NCQA Recognized Provider of quality diabetes care in your area: www.ncqa.org/dprp

To find an ADA Recognized Education Program in your area: Call 1-888-232-0822. www.diabetes.org/recognition/education.asp

To join the fight to increase funding for diabetes research, end discrimination, and improve insurance coverage: Call 1-800-342-2383. www.diabetes.org/advocacy

To find out how you can get involved with the programs in your community: Call 1-800-342-2383. See below for program Web addresses.

- *American Diabetes Month:* Educational activities aimed at those diagnosed with diabetes—month of November. www.diabetes.org/ADM
- *American Diabetes Alert:* Annual public awareness campaign to find the undiagnosed—held the fourth Tuesday in March. www.diabetes.org/alert
- *The Diabetes Assistance & Resources Program (DAR):* Diabetes awareness program targeted to the Latino community. www.diabetes.org/DAR
- *African American Program:* Diabetes awareness program targeted to the African American community. www.diabetes.org/africanamerican
- *Awakening the Spirit: Pathways to Diabetes Prevention & Control:* Diabetes awareness program targeted to the Native American community. www.diabetes.org/awakening

To find out about an important research project regarding type 2 diabetes: www.diabetes.org/ada/research.asp

To obtain information on making a planned gift or charitable bequest: Call 1-888-700-7029. www.diabetes.org/ada/plan.asp

To make a donation or memorial contribution: Call 1-800-342-2383. www.diabetes.org/ada/cont.asp